Debbie Flint

TILL
THE
FAT
LADY
SLIMS

2017 Edition

**Find out
how Debbie broke free
from the habits
of a lifetime.**

First published by the author in 2002; revised and updated January 2017

Published 2017 by Choc Lit Publishing – Non Fiction
Choc Lit Limited
Penrose House, Crawley Drive,
Camberley, Surrey GU15 2AB, UK

A CIP catalogue record for this book is available
from the British Library

ISBN 978-1-78189-333-3

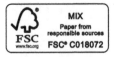

MIX
Paper from
responsible sources
FSC® C018072

Printed and bound by Clays Ltd

TILL
THE
FAT
LADY
SLIMS

2017 Edition

*With the utmost gratitude and big hugs to all the lovely
friends and relations and Freedom Eaters out there who
have all made this such a 'must-have' on their weight
loss journey. For all the fabulous new testimonials since I
wrote the original* Till the Fat Lady Slims *book in 2001,
through the subsequent updated version 2.0 and companion
book 3.0, and via the superb Facebook support groups of the
same name, thanks to you all. And to Choc Lit Publishing
for identifying the need for this more autobiographical
update, I salute you and thank you for all your support.*

DISCLAIMER

Please note – this book attempts to provide guidance for the understanding of natural eating. It is not, in any way, shape or form, a medical manual or a guide to treatment. If you think you may have a medical problem, you must see your medical practitioner. Nutritional needs are different from one person to another, and from one situation to another, including differences in gender, age and general health. Therefore you must use this book as a means of helping you make informed decisions about your dietary regime.

The author of this book is not a medical professional. Her aim is not to dispense any medical advice, directly or indirectly, regarding any technique mentioned in this book. You must always check with your medical practitioner before you start on any regime mentioned or described in this book. This book is not a substitute for any treatment prescribed by your doctor. The aim is to give you, the reader, general information, based on the author's own experience, to help you in your search for freedom from the eternal diet/gain weight cycle.

The author and publisher cannot be held responsible for actions that may be taken by a reader as a result of reliance on the information contained in this book, which are taken entirely at the reader's own risk.

Contents

Where it all Began

In 1999 Debbie Flint was working at QVC, the Shopping Channel, married with two children, and 35lb overweight.

This is the story of how she adopted a natural way of eating which she discovered whilst at QVC. She hadn't always been so overweight, but stressful life events and children, plus a marriage breakdown had taken their toll. Debbie originally trained as an accountant, and took a business degree at the London School of Economics before entering the world of television and radio. Having started her broadcasting career in radio, she became the first female presenter in the Children's BBC Broom Cupboard. That was followed by marriage, the arrival of her two children, stints on BBC Daytime TV, Living TV and ten years with Children's SSVC TV Forces' Television. In 1998 Debbie returned to BBC1 to host her own game show, *Meet the Challenge*, when she was nearly at her heaviest and feeling desperate for a permanent solution.

▶ *In 1999, Freedom Eating changed everything*

A QVC book and tape pack from Vikki Hansen and Shawn Goodman about the method of natural weight loss struck a chord and she not only started to lose weight, she stopped bingeing for good. But new science about hydration and hunger hormones meant giving it her own spin when, having used the system to change her life, and due to viewers' requests, Vikki and Shawn asked her to write her own version. This led to the 2002 original, *Till the Fat Lady Slims*.

Debbie then went on to spend nine years away from QVC before returning in 2009. In 2014 a new regular well-being show called *Back to You* put the focus squarely on how Debbie had lost weight and the updated *Till the Fat Lady Slims 2.0 – the 'When' Diet* was born, featuring the bitter truth about sugar addiction and other key information. Companion Book 3.0 brought in references to gut bacteria and the microbiome, the Inner Chimp and introduced the six guises of Freedom Eaters, identifying crucial differences in how we all regard dieting. She also set up the highly successful online support group 'Till the Fat Lady Slims' with a Facebook group and page, and started receiving many, many testimonials from those who had adopted the Freedom Eating system like a long lost friend. These feature on www.tillthefatladyslims.com.

Debbie says, 'In all my years of seeing thousands of products on Shopping TV, none had as much impact on me as the **Freedom Eating** pack – it may sound clichéd but it literally changed my life. Without it, I'd have had a return to binge-eating and massive weight gain. Instead, I've managed to stop bingeing forever – and regain a more healthy relationship with food.'

Having been asked for a more in-depth autobiographical version, Debbie is pleased to bring you this new book.

More than anything else, when new readers uncover the knowledge within these pages, they discover that what happened to Debbie echoes their own experiences:

> *'I could have been reading about myself … It made me cry, it resonated with me completely … I thought I was the only one, it's so good to know I'm not alone.'*

You're not alone. Debbie is there with you. Read this, the story of her Freedom Eating journey, join her online support system, and let her know how you get on, as she is always interested and learning from you, as much as you are from her.

Nowadays, Debbie Flint is happily writing novels, living with her 'flabradors' (fat Labradors) and continuing her QVC career. Her two grown-up children, Lauren and Bradley, are happily settled with their partners and thankfully have never had a life ruled by food.

This book features Debbie Flint's own story in more detail and with updated references plus:

- Debbie's story in-depth.
- A 'how to' section at the back, summarising the key principles of Freedom Eating and explaining in detail how to adopt it yourself, including using the 'When' Diet alongside any traditional diet – ANY.
- How different personalities can use Freedom Eating in different ways, to fit in with their own preferences for losing weight.
- Testimonials from successful members of the TTFLS gang.
- Further reading and more resources.
- How to keep in touch and join in the support groups.

Baby Steps

This book is designed to be read, and re-read, on a regular basis to help you adjust to the new patterns of behaviour. Please note the changes will take time, for most people.

Sometimes people fall by 'the wayside' as part of the journey – well that's okay too, and Debbie will explain how to deal with 'the wayside' later in the book.

This was me in 1999 ...

There's this woman who is the same as countless others of the same age. Always said she'd be different. Always knew she'd achieve something special in her life; whether a superstar career girl, mother, friend, lover or, naturally, a brilliant combination of all those. And she will do it – she has no doubt – one day. But first she just has to lose some weight. She's been saying it for some time now. In fact, trying to get a grip on the whole personal lifestyle thing. If she can – no – when she can do this, everything will be perfect. Everything will fall into place. Everything will start to happen.

Others like her have been saying it for years. And no one's ever contradicted her or made her think anything's amiss with her plan. Partly because she doesn't really discuss it all openly, just the dieting bit, and for many of them, that's accepted logic anyway: everyone diets, don't they? In fact, everywhere she looks there's only reinforcement for her philosophy – from her friends and family, from all the knowledge at her fingertips, from the media, from those perfect examples of 'before and after' that magazine and newspapers frequently publish. They all say the same thing – the weight will go when she stops eating so much of the wrong thing – whatever 'wrong thing' is in vogue right now. When she cuts back on calories, or fat grams, carbohydrates or points, units or whatever – carefully counting and controlling. Each new type of diet comes and goes, but there's always the next one. Yes, when she finds a diet plan that works, when she's 'good' and 'good' permanently – that's when it will all fall off and life can really begin again.

And she knows what it feels like to be 'good' – on the rare occasion she can call herself that, she's counting things, depriving and controlling – and maybe exercising consistently. That's good. Oh, and not smoking, or drinking too much, or arguing, or crying too often, or neglecting her friends/family/career – if she's really honest, that's really being 'good'. But it has to start with the right diet. And she knows that one day, in fact, one day soon, she'll be good all the time. After this next bad phase, in fact, right after it. NEXT TIME everything will work out. Isn't it always the way? So she'll just get over this bad phase, and happy days will be just around the corner, because only when she's good all the time is she allowed to be happy. But staying good all the time is so hard. Oh she's convinced herself that next time it'll last, she'll get it right, but in truth, she's never stayed good all the time.

She knows it's really her fault, she knows the rules and she's the one who's broken them, so *she's* the one to blame – not *the rules*. You're 'bad'. And you just need to be good – all the time – and then everything will fall into place. But right now, as you read this, she's just in one of her bad phases. It'll pass.

Of course there are other options – the get slim quick products and ideas and fads. If she did those successfully, followed yet another set of rules then those options would bring her happiness sooner. Cabbage soup every day, eat only protein, take these tablets, use that lotion, this machine – all the time. Yes, she could use those solutions, follow them thoroughly and be good at them, too – *all the time*. But she doesn't. So the half-finished tubs of pills and potions are still in the cabinet. The half-read books are still by the bed. The machine's back in its box (or loaned to a friend – Good Samaritan, right?) The exercise routine lasted a little while, then she found she ran out of time each day. The 'choose this not that', 'eat now not then' diet was too boring/difficult/tasteless/expensive/anti–social, so it, too, went by the wayside. Eventually, in the scheme of things, she's become a font of all knowledge – she knows the rules, but she *doesn't follow them*. Why not? Well, *no way* was it the diet's/tablet's/potion's/machine's/regime's/book's fault. Of course not, 'cos they all worked – for a while. So they must work – it's just they did not work for her. Because *she's to blame*. Of course! Because she didn't do it right – she couldn't be good – *all the time*.

Well, what if there was a different kind of 'good all the time', and it was easy? And it meant that over time you would lose the weight, and therefore get the life you're meant to have, and you could achieve the ultimate goal – to be happy every day.

▶ *It's called Freedom Eating.*

It's not a fancy technique or a passing phase – it's how slim people live and it's just going back to basics. What your body's been trying to tell you for all those years, through all those rules your brain introduced, through all the socialisation concerning food deprivation and control you've learned along the way. This is how you start listening to your body all over again. It's how to reclaim your right to be happy. This is the way you should be naturally – the way some people are – the way slim people are. But not you. Not yet.

But *you can be*. And it all begins with reclaiming your natural birthright to be slim. It's as natural as breathing. It's what your body was designed for. And the first step is Freedom Eating. If you read and re-read this book, and introduce it to your life, you can break free from Food Prison forever, and become that person you've kept on hold for years.

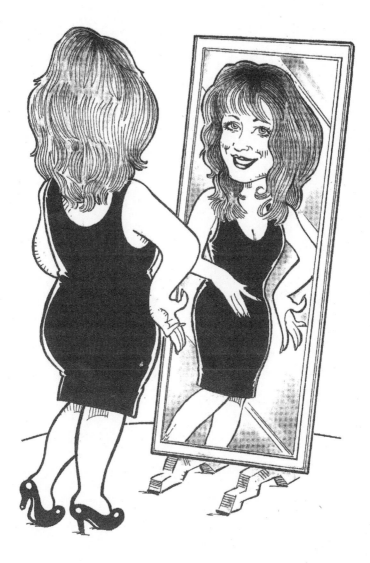

What do YOU see...?

From the Creators of
The Seven Secrets of Slim People

When we first met Debbie, she was the top performing host at QVC, UK, and we were presenting our product, The Seven Secrets of Slim People, *containing the principles of our original version of Freedom Eating, a non-diet weight loss program, based on all we had learned to that point. Debbie had started dabbling with Freedom Eating since the previous time we had been on QVC and was steadily and easily losing weight. In fact, Debbie would do each show with us with a carefully balanced tower of lard bricks stationed next to her chair. She would command the cameras to zoom into the pile of lard bricks. 'Each brick represents one pound of fat that I've lost on Freedom Eating,' she said, totalling, at that time 22 pounds. Today, of course, it's much more weight than that. Debbie's success with Freedom Eating inspired many of her loyal QVC followers to try it. Within a couple of weeks of our QVC shows with Debbie hosting us for the first time, we were swamped with letters from thrilled women whose lives were being changed by Freedom Eating. Debbie's belief in – and experience with – the Freedom Eating approach has single-handedly influenced thousands and thousands of women to follow in her footsteps in the UK. Finally, Debbie has decided to tell her own story. And what a story it is!*

One we all can relate to. You too will be inspired as you share in her ups and downs on the way to getting freedom with food and her ideal body. Freedom Eating began in the United States in 1986 when we tried to discover the secrets of becoming 'naturally slim'. To do this, we observed how naturally slim people ate and then copied their behaviours. As a result, we each lost over three stone, and have kept it off for years, without dieting at all.

And now, we thank you, Debbie, for sharing your powerful story with the world.

Vikki Hansen and Shawn Goodman, authors of
The Seven Secrets of Slim People and creators of
the original Freedom Eating system

Part One

1. In the World of the Fat

How long have you lived like this?
Were you as bad as me?

Surely someone who gets up in the
middle of the night to rake the bin
for leftovers can't be normal ...

It was 1984. I was twenty-two. Guests had come and gone and now the urges began. The spaghetti bolognaise wasn't so tempting, but skinny Jackie's barely touched jacket potato – still squashy with melted butter – was calling my name, loud. So as usual I replied, fished it out of the bin, and had a couple of minutes of heaven, devouring it alone in the dark. No one would know, no one would see, so it would all be okay, right? Except that it was *never* okay, and it was never enough. Afterwards, there was always that empty hole inside still waiting to be filled – a hole that not even the congealed, cold spag bol could touch. But I had to find out, just in case. After all, this time was the Very Last Time, wasn't it? The diet starts again tomorrow, and this time I'll stick to it. *Sound familiar?*

Yup, that was me. And at that time, *and* for most of the ten years before that, I considered myself to have a weight problem. But I didn't, not at the start anyway. I was just a normal kid with a few podgy bits. But no one convinced me that I didn't need to think I had this weight problem and I watched adults around me and their dieting behaviour. And I obeyed the commands to finish the plate and treat sugary treats as reward and comfort. So it became a food problem. Which became a big problem once I got into my own house, living all on my own.

I could do what I wanted, when I wanted, with whom I wanted, and eat all the leftovers the morning after. And all the while I'd be going on every diet under the sun to try to lose the weight: The F-plan diet, the cabbage diet, the fasting diet, the hi-carb diet, the low-carb diet, the high protein diet, the detox diet, the Beverly Hills diet, and the seafood diet. Yes, some nights even Terry the Jolly Lodger was in danger if he sat still too long!

Each diet worked at the start, and then didn't. With every new fad, or 'technique', my search for that instant solution was running out of options and none of them worked permanently. In fact, the only thing I achieved was a weight loss yo–yo that damaged my self-esteem, annihilated my self-image, and set in motion a downward spiral of abstaining and bingeing punctuated by the 'lose a few, gain a few more' pattern we all know so well, plus a long-running series of dreams about missing out on food. How was I to know it would take another fifteen years before I came across a solution so powerful, it has literally transformed people's lives?

Nowadays, I look back on those times with mixed emotions. Independence brings with it a greater cost than many a trainee grown-up realises. I paid my dues in comfort eating. The thing is, the comfort only lasted as long as each mouthful, and, on and off, I've gone through life dipping in and out of that safe habit place whenever the occasion arose, without quite knowing why I was there, or how to get back out again. Until the year when it all became clear.

At the time of starting the original version of *Till the Fat Lady Slims*, early 2000, I was a happily married busy career-type thirty-something. Two pregnancies made me a mother of two great kids, so now the fat is underneath a floppy belly and stretch marks. I'm a happy soul and most of the time the food problem is always played down, right? Apart from the occasional domestic crisis, or when there was too much month left at the end of the money again. Just like with everyone else, overdraft one, savings zero. Funny how each overdraft crisis was somehow temporarily cured with a chocolate biscuit or a bag of crisps. Still, a year after having my second baby I had managed to get back down to a good weight for me – 10st 5lb – positively slim for me. And why? Because – ah – let me recall. I was busy with my beloved, short-lived job as showbiz reporter on BSB. Anyone remember the 'squarials' back in 1990? Well, if you had one, you could have watched me on *31 West*. Full timetable, empty belly, happy bunny.

But all good things come to an end (thanks Rupert Murdoch), and the redundancies came, mine and my husband's, and then my dad died, and then the new shopping channel job started. Shift work, perpetual mother's guilt, something missing at home, never-ending treadmill, not enough love and too much angst. I was a bit of a nervous wreck one Christmas – crying whilst wrapping the presents and then going in for my shifts at QVC. It was just eighteen months after the launch of the fledgling shopping channel and it was doing well and I loved it. Plus I was strong, wasn't I? So without sharing my depression with anyone, I convinced myself The Man wasn't having affairs, pulled my socks up, went back to the grindstone at work, suffered more mother's guilt, and had one too many all-inclusive holidays and the weight piled on.

My quest for the solution turned a major milestone when I came across the programme called Freedom Eating in *The Seven Secrets of Slim People* in 1999 with guests Shawn and Vicky on QVC – and I haven't looked back since.

▶ *When the student is ready*

Little did people realise it but by the spring of 1999 I topped the scales at nearly thirteen stone – over 180lbs, and at 5′4″ – that is not good. The scales don't lie. They hate you, but you can't ignore their self-righteous proclamation that you've been a gut-bucket. You know it anyway, of course. I knew I'd been gaining at the rate of three or four pounds every six months since I had my 'bit of a wreck' thing roughly four years before. Quite an impressive feat, to hide the lot beneath designer clothes. Ever bigger ones, admittedly. Holiday shopping at Easter and I couldn't even get into size sixteen white pedal pushers – oh bugger.

My first size eighteens.

A fitted, tailored TV wardrobe had always made it too easy to hide the extra inches. Slip into a tailored jacket as well as, thank you God, Lycra bootleg trousers, and voila! The acceptable shape of TV shopping – just. I swear if I wasn't constantly 'on show', I'd have been a size twenty-eight by that point. Acceptable until those keep-fit hours started to become less of a challenge and more of an occasion to get totally stressed out.

I really was well and truly overweight by now. In an hour of selling keep fit stuff, I'd do a few exercises, then get off and let the guest instructor 'show us all how you do the next bit'. Then one day I just couldn't push myself up on the incline-bench-pulley thing, made a joke out of it with lots of grunting and heaving and joking and laughing. *Ha-ha, funny fat lady*. But I felt bloody frustrated, and didn't my fellow presenter, Paul, make a meal out of it as only a skinny can! What could I do but join in? So they just did it more.

Fatty jokes had become a regular part of my repertoire, and I must say – the 10lb bars of chocolate we were selling, or the set of two rich, moist fruit-cakes-in-a-tin, or the vertical roaster hours were crying out to be 'Debbie-fied'. Other show hosts mentioned my name in the same sentence as delicious food a little too often, and I began to truly start seeing myself as a 'fat person'.

– *'I have to go easy with the butt toner – it takes three minutes for my backside to stop wobbling.'*
– *'I'm just saving this crispy chicken skin for Debbie – I know she likes that.'*
– *'Now, to demonstrate this cleaner I've just made a big chocolatey mess on the carpet, good job Debbie's not around – she'd want to eat it.'*

You know the routine, and I must admit it was getting me down big time, and I knew I had to do something about it. But I love food – always have, and me and diets just never got on. I'd go on a diet, then come off a diet. I don't drink, smoke, gamble or a whole lot else and food was my panacea. The answer to everything. A crutch in good times and bad. You're lonely, you eat, you're angry, you eat, you're happy, let's go have a meal at the 'all-you-can eat' carvery and celebrate. It's a special occasion, you eat, you can always go back on the diet tomorrow. Yes, I'd think, I might as well make the most of it tonight and stuff myself because tomorrow all this will be once more out of bounds. We've all done that, haven't we? I'd had more Last Suppers than normal dinners.

The roots were in my childhood, I know it, and so was the accompanying fear of deprivation, fear of being hungry – panic, in fact – at being hungry, instead of just realising that it's a normal body function and ties in with the hormones that control when to stop. But what did it matter what my body said? My brain told me it was time to eat. Lunchtime, breaktime, anytime it was 'special' food, or 'free'. That's why the diets never worked. I already looked at food in a totally unnatural way anyway.

> ► *My mind chose limited, rationed and denied mode.*
> *I was constantly in deprivation and control.*

No chance my body would win through that lot. Let alone all those years of giving out messages of famine to my body by crash dieting, by always looking for the quick fix, making it lower my metabolism year on year with each diet. One of the most amazing facts discovered during learning about Freedom Eating for me was the study involving adults with normal appetites who were forced to go on diets. They actually automatically put on weight long-term as a result of consistently denying the body what it needed. Their metabolic rate had slowed down to accommodate this new situation of food sparseness, and they all had eating problems thereafter. The others who were given more food than they usually ate actually found their metabolisms also adjusted after a substantial time, and coped with all the extra food, and stayed higher thereafter.[1]

Being 'bad' is par for the course of a dieter's life, isn't it? And beating yourself up about it for the rest of the day is normal, isn't it? When the truth is, there's no 'good' or 'bad' behaviour surrounding food, there's 'just what the body wants,' 'what it doesn't want,' and crucially, '*when* to eat it'. And believe it or not, you can rediscover how to make use of this in order to get slim and stay there, whilst – amazingly – really having a good time enjoying your food and eating all your favourites whenever you're hungry. Unbelievable? Or achievable heaven?

▶ *Eureka*

Imagine your food prison. You're in a big cage. No one knows it's there except you. The bars of this cage are the barriers that keep you from ever feeling 'normal' around food. You've been in this cage for so long, you think there is no key. The wrong rules keep you inside this prison. Do these still govern your life?

– *'You must finish your plate even if you feel stuffed.'*
– *'You must have your vegetables then you can have some pudding.'*
– *'You're too slow – eat faster.'*
– *'You can't have cheese on top – it's fattening.'*
– *'Look at your bum – it's 'cos of all those sweets you keep eating.'*
– *'Don't have more bread – you won't eat your main course.'*

And so, so many more.

These rules help keep you in this prison. They are the bars through which you view the world and make your decisions surrounding every scrap of food that passes your lips. Now imagine someone comes along one day; a white knight on a charger, and declares that all these rules, which you've lived by for so long, inherited or made up for yourself, just ... don't count. They aren't true, and you can ignore them. He unlocks the key to your prison and lets you out. *Oh my God. So this is where the slim people live!*

Want all those things you've been depriving yourself of for so long, all those things that skinnies have all the time – have them.

However, this is the crucial thing – the one condition – you only have it if your *body* really wants it. This book will help you distinguish what, when and how much, and contains new information helping to make sense of the body's signals and new resources with information on what can upset these crucial signals. How, for instance, fructose in sugar can override them. Back when I first learned Freedom Eating I just instinctively knew it, but since then a whole raft of new science has come to light backing this up. A calorie is truly not a calorie. New science throughout the 2010s proves this over and over again. Later on I give you some more information so you can go be your own project.

It's actually fun learning the process and getting to know your body, your best friend, all over again.

It equally feels like heaven to say 'yes' to some of the foods you thought were 'bad' – but you're only saying yes to eating that one food, right there, right then, for as long as it feels good. You'll learn how Freedom Eating is NOT saying yes to making it a full blown 'blow-out' just because you ate one biscuit too many or finished the kids' cake.

Or you might change your mind halfway through and stop, because you can.

But what you're not doing is saying yes to losing control for the rest of the day, and opening the doors to a tidal wave of overeating because you've stepped outside the prison and all its rules. So eat that food – without judgement – if you want it. And that's the next crucial pointer.

▶ *You only eat it for so long as your body wants it.*

You stop when your body is satisfied, not when you can't

breathe any more. Not when you're full up. Just doing what the body would do naturally if your mind, and society, had never interfered. The body is magic, it knows these things.

And what a relief it is once you acknowledge that.

And what about all those times you 'fill–up on vegetables'. Well, you don't have to, you know. Eat too much of any food and you'll put on weight. Eat at the wrong time, when you're not hungry, and your body will just put it into storage and convert it to fat on your hips. Eat loads of 'healthy' rice and vegetables all day long, till you are bursting, then go to sleep and you can become a Sumo wrestler! Why do so many dieters feel they have to fill themselves up by overeating vegetables? They may be only vegetables, they are really, really good for you – but why overeat them? Why overeat anything?

There is an important point to be noted here, and that is that there are many people who trust themselves so little, that the mere thought of listening to the body to make food choices brings them out in a slight panic. If you're a serial dieter or if you just don't believe true Freedom Eating can work for you, don't worry. There's a whole section later called 'the "When" Diet,' created in 2014 with the help of my sister, an ex-slimming club leader. Ideal if you feel safe around traditional diets, and want to ease yourself into all this freedom stuff gradually; then don't worry, you can give yourself the freedom to do it that way. The most important thing is to feel comfortable and happy with it, and if you're too scared to go the whole hog immediately, then introduce it step-by-step – as recommended later in this book.

But just do it, if you can, even if you stay at step one for a year. Because long term, it will be better for you than what's been happening in your life so far, otherwise, why would you be reading this book? Don't be frightened.

Yes, unlearning the beliefs you've had for donkeys' years will be a little scary at first, so give yourself permission to try it stage by stage, and enjoy the process. There are so many little exciting discoveries that make it all worthwhile. I've been making discoveries continuously – little 'Aha's' – some of which I write about in this book for the first time. You just have to understand what your own discoveries are.

▶ *Unlearning.*

Ever seen a baby turn its head and refuse to take any more bottle? It's had enough, and it stops eating. It just stops. You never force a baby to eat more, do you? Force the bottle back in its mouth? No! So why do it with a toddler? Or a teenager, or an adult? If we hadn't been brainwashed over the years, throughout our childhood and adolescence and young adulthood and old adulthood, we'd never have lost that response to stop when the body is satisfied. But it's not too late to get it back. Just think about it and you've got to admit it's true. We just need to unlearn all the 'manual overrides' from years and years of deprivation and control.

▶ *Deprivation and control – yuk.*

Without deprivation and control, we'd be exactly how we were when we were born – with a specially evolved, perfect eating mechanism you can always trust to gauge exactly what to eat, and for how long, and when. It's called your body, and deep down within the confusion and desperation and fear, it's waiting. Just waiting to be handed back the keys to your mouth. Funnily enough, studies on babies' eating habits showed that even when some were fed on a more low-fat formula, their bodies automatically knew they needed to consume more, whilst they drank less if it was a richer concentration.

There is categorically no doubt that you *can* trust your body. Its innate, inbuilt, fundamentally automatic mechanisms for getting you what you need, when you need it, are lying dormant inside you, and what fun to bring them out of hibernation and into full use again. Make it fun – listen to your body – without judgement. Because being judgemental, being critical of yourself, is the password to another Last Supper.

Psssst! Hey, prisoner, here's an escape route for you – keep it to yourself though – only the skinnies know about this one! It's this: if you overeat one time, it's fine. 'What do you mean, fine? How can it possibly be fine? I've been bad.' No actually, skinnies will do what you call 'bad' things all the time. Want to be one of them? Well, how about this – just observe.

▶ *Don't judge.*

Don't beat yourself up about it. If you want some chocolate – really genuinely want it, not in your head but in your body, have it. If you overeat a little, and pretty soon it'll only ever be a little, say to yourself – 'Interesting, I wonder why I did that,' and then just get on with your life.

Don't waste any more time thinking about it, deliberating on what to do next, how to punish yourself for being such a terrible person, or generally being a food prisoner.

Act like a slim person – just move on. I wish someone had told me this all those years ago. When I first realised I was truly fat.

▶ *Is this you? This used to be my mantra – was it yours?*

It's when you look at the photo and don't recognise yourself. When you see your inner self in the mirror because the external version is too alien to accept. When comfort eating is not just the solution, it's the beginning, the middle and the end of every day. That's when the fat lady has well and truly arrived. And you don't have to be outwardly 'fat' to have a fat lady take over your mind. How many of us hear someone we know saying, 'I'm too fat, I need to lose at least, ooh, five pounds,' and watch in stunned disbelief as they grip at a mere half an inch or so of paltry pudge around their middle, knowing that we'd win this game hands down with our three or four rolls of at least an inch or two each.

▶ *We're fat. We know it. We just don't know what to do about it.*

Well, for starters, how about looking into your past, at the behaviours society taught you, the rules and regulations you learned, the control and deprivation your mind lives its life by. All as a result of what we were told as we grew. There are people untouched by these habits. They are the slim people. The skinnies. The 'I can eat anything I want' brigade, who make our already inadequate self-image even more resentful and controlling and scared. We haven't a clue how they can leave one mouthful of a chocolate bar, or the last bite of a burger, or the final pea on their plate. Or how they've been known to skip a meal. How they can say they don't want any dessert. Or how they can resist the temptation to share that oozing creamy birthday cake one day, yet tuck into a whole half a packet of biscuits the next. Without ever seeming to put on a pound. Well, guess what? I've studied these slim people. And I've found out how. I've looked at what they do to stay at their ideal weight, whilst eating normally.

▶ *It's called Freedom Eating. And now you can do it too.*

The Seven Secrets of Slim People by Vikki Hansen and Shawn Goodman and the associated tape programme[2] from around 1998 helped thousands of people on both sides of the Atlantic to finally break free from food prison, to start living normal lives around food, and to gradually lose weight in the easy, enjoyable, favourite-food-filled process.

For me, having discovered it whilst at work at QVC UK, it meant turning the clock back ten years. Losing two and a half stone (35 pounds or so) naturally, and having my self-respect and dignity back. It's not a quick fix. It's not a temporary solution. It's not aided by tablets or injections or mad exercise regimes. It's not a guide to what to eat when, and how much it should measure. It's a practical, common sense step to permanent freedom from food prison. Freedom Eating. And whether you adjust to it gradually, step-by-step, starting off alongside your diet, or go the whole hog immediately, this method can be used by everybody. Absolutely everybody.

It'll free you up to be the person you deserve to be and bring you the body you were meant to have naturally, had you never interfered with it. Plus, it will affect those closest to you as they too emulate your behaviour. Yes, Freedom Eating means happier, slimmer kids too.

So what is Freedom Eating?

In a nutshell it's how slim people eat:

- Listen to your body – it knows best.
- Drink lots of water if you're not sure. You might be thirsty rather than hungry.
- Eat when your body is ready – when you are at hunger level six (I'll explain more later).
- Do nothing else while you eat. Nothing. Concentrate on the food and give it your full attention.
- Think carefully about WHAT to eat, knowing nothing is out of bounds as long as it's what your BODY wants, not your mind. (Alongside any traditional diet you choose from your list of foods, but still choose the best fit for that moment.)
- Eat only until satisfied (not full); this is crucial – usually about a fistful of food. Keep the rest till later.
- Watch out for the bliss point, that's what your body will give you when you've had the perfect amount of exactly the right food, at the right time.
- Don't feel guilty if you go wrong – be kind to yourself. You're not 'bad' just learning.

- Observe afterwards how the meal makes your body feel and choose better next time. There is no 'wrong' just more accurate, or less accurate, choices.

Plus:
- Don't let others put you off – they'll gradually get used to the new you. Only you know what's best for you – or your body does. Baby steps are still steps. Get into 'perma habits' – what you do most, each day, defines who you are. Small changes are fine.
- The wayside is okay, just dust yourself off and get back in the swing at the very next mealtime, don't 'eat the cupboards empty' and think 'I'll start again tomorrow.' You've done that for years, so do this instead.

Full explanations are supplied throughout and in depth information in Part Two, but briefly here are the 'Super Six' Principles of Freedom Eating.

1. Don't eat until you are at 6 on the hunger scale.
2. Be accurate in what you choose – try to eat exactly what your body wants.
3. Pay full attention to your food when you eat.
4. Stop eating when satisfied and not when full.
5. Aim for the bliss point.
6. Examine the way your body feels afterwards.

So what do you say? Give it a go? The information you're about to discover doesn't work unless you use it. Like anything, there are things that will rest easily with your lifestyle, and there may be things that don't work for you initially. Just do whatever feels right for you. Once you start really understanding what your body wants – with food at first – you'll end up in a better place than you ever thought possible, and so will your family. It's the first step to Freedom Living – and that's a real eye-opener, I can tell you.

So if you love freedom and hate dieting, this is for you – if you've ever dreamed of that elusive, all-consuming freedom not to ever count another calorie, fat gram, carb unit or point, not to ever have to step on the scales to decide whether you're going to have a good or a bad day, and not to ever have to follow the strangling, restricting, uncomfortable rules you've been led to believe are the only ones available to you concerning food, read on. And if you like the 'safety' of following a plan, you can also use this system to benefit from easing yourself into Freedom Eating step-by-step. Eventually it will be your best friend, helping to avoid the patterns of self-sabotage that undo all the good work and make the weight go right back on again. In fact, once this incredibly enjoyable, easy system becomes habit, you'll never look back and you'll wonder how you ever 'unlearned' this natural way to be slim.

2. In the World of the Slim

The first steps to 'unlearning' all the
beliefs that have made you fat ...

There are certain facts we live with all our lives that we accept as gospel. But what if there are new facts? Facts that, once you discover them and accept that they really do work for you, can really make you start to feel at home in this new world where the slim people live. At certain 'times of the month', you may just need more food. Sometimes at certain times of the year, you may need less – in which case *don't* eat just because 'it's time to'. Or just because the family's about to eat. So? Just sit with them, with your food in front of you, and if you're not hungry, wait till you *are* and save it till later – why not? It's a good example to your kids too, if you need any more reasons! Later on when you're sufficiently hungry once more, it will taste better anyway. Then your body will be ready to digest, and not to store. It's important to say at this stage that I do full Freedom Eating, where the food world is my smorgasbord, and I can choose from anything. I'll explain later about how to use it whilst dieting, and also how different people respond in different ways. I've discovered, through years of dealing with different types of people, that there are different 'guises' of Freedom Eater. One of them will be just like you.

> ▸ *Full Freedom Eating to Break Free From Food*
> *Prison*

If you fancy a treat, pick your favourite food, the one that shouts at you – because that'll be your body telling you what nutrients it needs most at that time, if you listen carefully enough. (In recent years the groundbreaking new information about gut bacteria taught me exactly why that happens. See later.) And it won't always be the same. True, people who've always denied themselves certain things, for example, bacon, or raspberry milkshake, may find their bodies want *just* that for a while. But get enough and your body won't be shouting for it any more, and you'll move on from it. That's why, unlike with most diets, my own method is this – to fill your house with your *most* favourite things.

> ▶ *Oh no, now she's really gone mad!*

Are you thinking this – 'I know what I'm like if I have those foods in the house, I'll binge like crazy, and once I've started I just can't stop.' Or, 'If I even think about those foods, or smell them, I start to get sweaty palms because I know they're my downfall …'

Well, hear me out on this one, okay? There's a defined logic to this argument, which you won't fail to understand, and as long as you follow it, it will work – instead of endlessly repeating old habits – reliving your own bad eating history like groundhog day.

Here's the theory that makes full Freedom Eating work for me. If those 'danger foods' are there for the taking, your mind knows there's no shortage, and the craving for them will gradually go away. At that point, a mischievous 'being' inside you, called the Inner Chimp, is prevented from sliding into panic mode. (See later for more about this Inner Chimp.)

Tell yourself you *can* have one. Stop it being treasure. Choose to eat just that – eat it first – the next time you're hungry. Try it! Oh my God, it's a veritable gift from heaven that someone should even suggest this to you, but what if it's true? Try it! Say you *can* have it, and really, really mean it. Say, 'I can have it.' Go on, do it now, imagine that doughnut or toast with butter or full fat yogurt being in your mouth. Or whatever you really, really fancy. How lovely. 'Oh yes, yes, YES!' Meg Ryan will have nothing on you when this fabulous flavour-filled mouthful floods your taste buds. Take another bit, then another, and keep observing what it tastes like – what it feels like in your mouth, as you swallow. Keep going until you get the deep breath, indicating you are satisfied and it's time to stop. (See later for full explanation on how to tell exactly when to stop.) Maybe that Meg Ryan moment, from the film *When Harry Met Sally*, has subsided and the food that was so amazing just now, doesn't taste as gob-smackingly wonderful any more. Is that now? If so, then it's time to click in with the new decisions.

The New Decisions

– *'I don't have to finish it just because it's there.'*
– *'I don't have to eat all of it.'*
– *'I'm allowed to save the rest for later, and if my body still wants it when I'm next hungry, I can have it all over again. But if I don't, I won't.'*
– *'If my body really, really wants more right now, I can have it.'*
– *'If I'm not sure, I'll wait fifteen minutes, then assess it again.'*
– *'I must just listen to my body and go with what it's telling me.'*
– *'My body is giving me permission to go ahead and eat the forbidden foods, for a trade-off – I must take notice of it.'*
– *'I will not let it down. In return, I will listen to the signals.'*

Makes sense doesn't it? And what of your choices normally? When you're on yet another new regime, for instance? How many times during a diet do you eat things that you wouldn't touch with a bargepole normally? It's just that if someone says you 'cannot' have the nicer versions, then it makes you want them more. Been there? Know the place? Bought the T-shirt? Food prisoners live in that place. Permanently. Remember that other important escape route. Say, 'I can have it if my body really wants it, as much of it as my body wants till my tummy is pleasantly satisfied and physically doesn't want any more.' NOT 'Till I'm full, or till they're all gone, or till someone comes in and sees me.' Just till I'm 'satisfied'. Simple.

▶ *Liberation!*

Yes, it is really possible to suddenly transform your life and not have to abide by those binding, restrictive, negative, depressing, straightjacket beliefs you hear all the time – from yourself and others. It's a fabulous feeling, you wait till you try it.

▶ *Start listening to your body and not to your brain,*
  or to anyone else's brain for that matter.

That's what I did way back when. With a cynical eye, I must admit. Even though I listened to The Seven Secrets of Slim People avidly, and was very up for giving it a go, I still had that sceptical edge.

But as soon as I 'got' it, something clicked. You can do the same. Then you'll be on your way to Freedom Eating. It's so logical. Because if you always make your body eat diet food, even though it really wants just a little of the full-fat version, you'll probably feel totally frustrated after eating the low-fat alternative, you may even do what I used to do, and go through the lot, and still come back to the 'bad' one in the end. Then we just feel that we've let ourselves down again by 'giving in', don't we? In any case, low-fat is old hat, as recent headlines have shown. Think about the study using low-fat formula on babies – they just ate more of it. They naturally knew they didn't have what their bodies needed. The opposite of when a baby turns its head away – it knows when it's had enough, or not had enough. Hey, in life outside the prison, it's okay to have some of what you fancy – that old saying is never truer – but a little of what you fancy is almost certainly what you'll end up having if you allow your body to tell you when to stop. I'll say that again, because I've found it to be so true.

▶   *A LITTLE of what you fancy is almost certainly what you'll have if you truly listen to your body's signals.*

You only go into overdrive and finish the whole packet of chocolate chip cookies if your mind takes over and starts distorting what your body's trying to tell you, then you start feeling like a criminal for breaking 'The Rules'. If you can convince yourself it's all okay, and simply move on from each little misdemeanor, they'll be less and less frequent and that's what should happen. After all, you're not going to get this perfect from the outset, and you can congratulate yourself because you are finally on a path to permanent weight loss. If you find yourself wanting sugary things ALL the time and it never seems to hit the spot, and never gives you the true Meg Ryan moment, then maybe you're sugar addicted. (See later for how to deal with that.) Then you can get out of the way of your body's signals.

Trust in your body – it knows what path to take. Your mind doesn't. It only thinks it does after years of being in the pilot's seat. It's just like flying an aircraft; 90% of the time, a plane is off-course, but every little correction brings it back on line till in the end, it's right on target.[3] That's what it'll be like when you start listening to your body and letting it do what it does naturally, without your mind interfering. But first you have to help it along. Baby steps, remember? It doesn't happen overnight, but there are lots of little tips and extra guidelines here to help you give your body a chance to adjust. After all, you've been following these habits for years, right? So just like when you drive home and you go into automatic, and suddenly you've arrived, and you don't know how you got there? If you've followed that same route for years, it becomes ingrained in your psyche, biologically speaking: the electrical pathways in your brain are a well-trodden trail, and once you get going in the right direction, your body automatically takes over and knows which neuron connects to which and basically what to do next.

That's why you must be forgiving of yourself initially, whilst you scramble these old pathways, and take a refreshing new route at each key junction along the way. The more you get used to it, the more automatic the new way of eating will be in the end, and you'll be eating like a slim person. Establish new pathways and your mind will gradually let go of the old ones that made you fat. As it observes the transformation in your body, and in your being, and as you gradually shed the excess pounds left by overeating, your mind will learn to trust your body. You will instinctively know what you need to do, and, more importantly than anything else, what you *don't* need to do.

3. Ten Pounds of Lard

*Don't let the scales decide if you're going
to have a good day – throw them out!*

Do you know how heavy ten pounds is? Ten one-pound packs of lard. Ten cans of soup. Put it in a carrier bag, walk up the stairs with it. Try to run with it. When I first began using Freedom Eating I had the biggest revelation. I was around thirteen and a half stone and so frustrated and unhappy. I'd never been able to diet, as I say. Rather, I was the one who rebelled. Well, to be more accurate, my Inner Chimp did! (See later.) So sitting in a McDonald's near Hastings and watching the kids eat their food, having just enjoyed – really truly enjoyed for the first time in years – chips and a burger, I felt the deep breath and stopped. It was completely alien to me, as it may be to many of you. But keep at it, it will soon become as normal as breathing.

By November 1999, I'd lost ten pounds of lard, and two inches off my waist. I still had more than twice that to lose. How the hell did I get to be that heavy in the first place? It was still early days, but I'd been adjusting to what I discovered is right for me using my new-found Freedom Eating, and a useful kick-start I'll tell you about later. But, for the first time in my life, I was confident and there was no reason to think the weight loss would stop. Sure, there are ups and downs, but I was sure as hell not going to punish myself for a hiccup in what amounted to a mere solitary measurement of progress – and one which doesn't give you the full picture. Yes I'm talking about that chief offender, the scales. The Freedom Eating guide allows you to ignore the scales. I'll say it again.

▶ *Ignore the scales. Never own any again. I said never!*

You have full permission to go right ahead and walk straight by them. They no longer have the God-given right to set you up or knock you back for the rest of the day. They may cry out to be caressed by your 'plates of meat', but you shall fear not and resist their temptation because muscle is heavier than fat, and body weights fluctuate hour by hour, let alone day by day, so ignore them. The serial dieter weighs several times a day not just the once a week conventional wisdom recommends. What's the point of that? It's all just information in the end, but information doesn't change your life, unless you act on it, and incorporate it in a way that works for you. So ignore it, and as for the rest of the information that abounds and surrounds us in our daily fight against the flab, well, pick out what works for you and ignore the rest.

▶ *Begin Freedom Living too!*

You should definitely follow your instincts and do what's right for you personally, whether using the guidelines given here, or in any of the literature accompanying the numerous weight-loss clubs and magazines and books and videos and the rest.

I did, in fact, technically lose seven pounds once by counting points and doing Weight Watchers. I had been successfully knocking down the walls of my food prison with the embryonic months of Freedom Eating, but it was early days and I had an offer I thought I should take. It was September 1999, and Weight Watchers had offered to use me for PR purposes, and came to the QVC building in Battersea to sign me up to their programme. The carrot for doing it was possibly featuring in one of their pieces in *The Sun*. Shallow and obvious, but the truth. So I agreed. Me, agreeing to a diet. I should have known better. They sent a lovely lady called Jacqui to me every week, with a fab supply of chewy breakfast bars, and caramel sweets and fruit pastille things that gave me the 'runs' the day I over-ate them. But I followed the diet, and followed it … till I couldn't stand it any more!

Now I don't want to put off anyone from using slimming clubs if they really honestly work for you. Unlike the original Freedom Eating guide, I won't say 'never go', because I know a lot of people just don't ever think they can trust themselves enough to go it alone. You've been so used to getting guidance all your life that the mere thought of depending on your body's signals to choose what to eat, along with being given permission to eat all those things you've always thought of as 'forbidden' or 'sins', plus the idea of eating as much as you want, really blows your mind. If that's you, read this bit, but then make sure you read the new section later about the 'When' Diet, detailing how Freedom Eating works alongside any traditional diet – any. You just take the bits that work for you, and leave the rest out till you feel confident enough to tackle full on Freedom Eating. You won't be alone. (See the 'When' Diet section later and read about the 'Linda' guise of Freedom Eater – if you like diets you're probably a Linda too!)

Anyway, having started counting points with gusto, I was gradually getting completely hacked off with the counting, the limitation, the 'can have, can't have' mentality. The 'lose half a pound = good girl, gain half a pound = bad girl'. Oh my God, we're talking about half a pound here. It descended to the farcical when I was asked, 'Have you had a poo yet, that could make a difference.' Of course it would. Half a pound is ridiculous. I could put on half a pound and lose it again within a few hours. How can this be right, or good for me psychologically, to be measured by that and only that? Were we looking at percentage body fat? No. Even though there are some fab gadgets if you really want to do this measuring lark. No, we were just weighing me. For goodness sake, at least give yourself a chance by not making weight loss the only consideration in whether you've been 'good' or 'bad'. Fat content may have gone down, even though your actual weight has gone up. Look at inches, even! I think every weight loss class in the country – no, in the world – should be legally made to measure people by other factors, not just weight. Along those lines, my new

Facebook group established around 2014, encourages 'NSVs' – non-scales victories – from our members.

Anyway, needless to say, after a few weeks of the counting lark, my Inner Chimp was rebelling big time, my morale started taking a nosedive, and pretty soon, I was cheating on the 'What have I eaten this week' chart, and beating myself up all over again, having not done it for bloody ages. I was also exercising like a mad woman to try to account for those couple of extra points I'd consumed, and driving everyone up the wall. Oh, and – just a minor point – feeling depressed, obsessed, and stressed.

That's what conventional wisdom says is the right way to lose weight, is it? Well, you can keep it. The breaking point came at the end of October 1999 when we went away with the kids to a villa in Cyprus. Self-catering, so we made the trip to the supermarket to scour the place for loads of non-fat stuff. Remember this was in the old days before they realised that it's not low fat that's important; it's sugar that's worse. (See later.) In any case, the trip there was excruciating, for me and The Man, and the kids – who had depressingly also started to act differently around food as a result of my obsession again. Oh-oh. Danger. A couple of little secret binges and the old me started to re-emerge and I was frightened, and finally turning into a rat-bag of the first degree was the last straw. I couldn't do it to myself, I couldn't do it to the kids and I couldn't do it to The Man. So I made the decision to go back immediately to the safety of my beloved full-scale Freedom Eating, and by the time I got back home, Weight Watchers Jacqui was proud to announce that I'd actually lost a pound.

▶ *I'd lost a pound.*

Now had I stayed on Weight Watchers, I'd have absolutely started bingeing and dieting, bingeing and dieting and would have gained the whole seven pounds back again, started making excuses why I couldn't make the weigh-in that week, and eventually given up, chiding myself for being a loser, a failure, and feeling ostracised from all the other goody-goodies who'd all lost weight that week but I hadn't. Sound familiar? It should. Apparently, the great majority – and it's been quoted at over 90% – of the weight lost through dieting and slimming clubs is regained within a few years. So why do people still go? Because 80% of the publicity for these places is generated by the 20% of the people who have lost, or are currently losing, weight. We've all been privy to the conversations where our friends have boasted about that week's successful weigh-in. But do they often speak of the weeks where they put it on? No. The PR machine churns out success story after success story, prompting more and more troubled fatties to join up. But how many follow-up stories do we hear of? How many times do they revisit their champions from previous years? You get my point.

Now there are some exceptions to all this, maybe you're one of them – one of the few who have used a slimming club once to permanently lose weight, but the likelihood is that type of person hasn't spent a lifetime yo–yo dieting without success, and buggered up their metabolism completely in the process. Or quietly binged and felt so ashamed they daren't own up to anyone – including themselves. Often that type of person is a one-off dieter – and it works. If that isn't you, and it certainly wasn't this fatty, well forget it! If you say, 'But hang on a minute, Debbie, those clubs have always worked for me in the past, every time I go back there I always lose the weight.' Hey, why the need to go back in the first place? It angers me because a fortune is spent treating the symptom and not the cause of weight gain. It's like trying to get someone to learn Chinese by showing them a pretty pattern on a page and telling them what sound to make when they see it, hey presto, you're 'speaking Chinese'. It works, till you forget what you were taught, become bored with the same old symbols, don't feel you're progressing, or just lapse back into speaking the same old language you're used to because you've done it for years. And with this system, including the online support group and resources, you're never on your own and you never need to get bored. That's my take on such things anyway. If you love diets, and have specific reasons for going to diet clubs, that's fine too – you have to do what's right for YOU.

If you don't understand what's going on, the weight loss will never be permanent. And in this updated version of my original *Till the Fat Lady Slims*, I share with you the fascinating discoveries about the body, which have helped to explain a system I've been using since 1999. I always knew they worked, just not why. Well, stand by to be amazed when I tell you later.

I tried to learn Greek once, with an audio tape and nothing visual. It lasted about as long as the holiday, but the French I got to know at school, and the German, even though I only did it for two years, sticks with me to a certain extent to this day because we learned about what the verb was, how to conjugate it, what the genders are, how to use them, what the tenses are, and how they fit in. We understood it, so it stayed with us. And so it will be with Freedom Eating. Once you understand it, you'll wonder how you lost touch with it for all those years. It's so easy, it's so bloody enjoyable, so logical, feels so good, you'll be hard-pressed not to go back to it time and time again, after every temptation to stray. Some people will never stray – it'll be as natural once more as breathing. For others, like me, who live their lives on an improvement crusade, and are willing to go back to the hard work of finding other alternatives, going back to choosing with the brain not the body, listening to current thinking about various eating fads, or trying to abstain from certain foods, it'll be something to which you will always return with open arms at the end of a difficult journey, like coming back home at the end of the wars.

So diet if you must, but follow the 'When' Diet – which incorporates most of the principles of Freedom Eating at the same time – and you'll be well on the way to a more natural way of eating. The body's own way – the way we were born – the way our body wants to eat if we only give it the chance. Think, do I really want it? Does my BODY really want it? How will it feel afterwards? Do I really want more of it? Can I feel the food in my stomach yet? Stop if you can, once you're satisfied. And then gradually work towards trusting your own body once more. Give it back the control and you'll never need to suffer the indignities of being one of the 'bad girls' and feeling that old 'naughty little girl panic' as the slimming class begins to lose its shine once more.

Lecture over! Haha!

So having lost the seven pounds with the slimming club, I have to add that you and I both know what would have normally happened at that point had I not gone back to Freedom Eating. Another few weeks passed and I reached the ten pound stage. This was ten pounds lost since the initial Weight Watchers weigh in, mind you, 12st 6lb. I have to say I was more than that originally, but I'd been scared to get on the scales for a long time. I'd not measured the loss in between starting Freedom Eating and suffering the diversion of counting stuff, and going back to deprivation and control. But if you'd seen some of the photos, notably the one with Tony Robbins, the US Success Coach, when I hosted one of his hours in November 1998, you'd be shocked at the size of my face. And, bless his rapport techniques, even then he told me, 'your husband's a lucky man'. (If only the husband – now the ex-husband – thought that, haha!)

So I couldn't be certain, but I know by appearance and past experience, I was over 13 stone back then – around 13st 4lb. I'd looked that way once before in my life – about the time of the spaghetti bolognaise in the dustbin scenario – and I hated myself. Thank God for Freedom Eating, it took me down to 12st 6lb in around four months.

4. Do What I Do

*Water, and the body's
many cries for help.*

Okay, having worked with this system for so long, and having noted some omissions, this book contains my own updated version of Freedom Eating. There are some things I'd like to recommend in addition to the original Freedom Eating guidelines, and the first involves drinking water. Do it. There, I've said it. If I could get everyone to drink more water, even if it's just ordinary water, I'd be happy. But now I have to say once more that you should do what feels right for you and your body. But as far as water is concerned, just try it for a while for me and see. Yes, drink water, two to three litres a day is recommended, more accurately, drink half your bodyweight (measured in pounds,) in ounces of water. For example, if you're 140lb (10 stone) then drink 70 ounces per day (16 fl oz is about 500ml). More and more is being discovered about how good it is to be fully hydrated. So I drank more water, and I exercised. I'm a firm believer in it, and if you are too, then great. But it's your decision, you do what's right for you. The same thing goes with exercise.

Generally speaking, we have all known for years what we should be doing, as regards 'moving more' and it's still the case. Don't get me wrong, what's best for your body is definitely to do some exercise as well, but you don't need to go mad! If you combine healthy eating with exercise, as many people do by just changing their lifestyle rather than treating it all as a temporary and drastic measure, you'll help yourself to stay younger longer, as well as helping your metabolism. I had a dog, Holly, born in June 1999 and she helped to give me a good forty-five minutes brisk walk every day, which did wonders for my fitness and energy levels, my ability to walk upstairs without getting out of breath and my sense of well-being and being able to cope with those fitness hours on QVC once again!

Whatever exercise works for you, I personally recommend you do some, (check with your GP if you're unsure what type to go for), but walking, or a treadmill if you can't get out, is as good a place as any to start. Get a Fitbit or pedometer – ten thousand steps a day is a superb target to aim for. Or whatever is right for you. Find something you enjoy, build it up gradually, but don't wear yourself out or give yourself a headache by doing too much too quickly and maybe you'll be able to feel little but consistent improvement over the weeks and months. Just get it into your life, somehow, even a few minutes a day, then build up from there. HIIT (High Intensity Interval Training) exercise is in the headlines again and involves less effort for more benefits; using a thing called the Bodyblade is my favourite type of HIIT routine – google it. Again, listen to your body, and if it hurts, you're not doing it right!

But exercise on its own is not the best way to use up the calories you've just eaten. You need to do half an hour's aerobic work-out to allow yourself a Mars bar, or thereabouts, so you'd have to do some serious sweating or heavy physical work to balance out a typical huge eating binge. And any binge is by definition too much for your body's natural needs, so think seriously about the Freedom Eating guidelines and start practising Freedom Living if you also find yourself on the inside of an exercise prison, not just a food prison. (However if bingeing is top of your list, turn to the back section about Binge Management.)

How many people, especially guys, have you known, who believe the way to being slimmer is to work out all hours? Vikki Hansen's hubby used to work out, up to six hours a day, in order to live life as a Grade A Gutbucket. He was fit, not fat, renowned for finishing off everyone else's leftovers, consuming mammoth portions and generally living in a different kind of prison – rules, rules, bloody rules. He believed that it would 'turn to fat' if he ever gave himself a breather and stopped the punishing exercise ritual. God forbid he should listen to his body's food needs and just maybe one day try not eating huge amounts.

If you live with someone like that in your life, then there's even more reason why this programme will be a godsend. Imagine if he or she could stop and just consider the idea that they actually didn't have to manically stick to their training schedule if they just ate what their body wants and not what they think it wants. To not have to dutifully slave over a hot treadmill for a couple of hours a day? Wow! It's liberation of a whole different kind.

I used to help my dad with his contract cleaning business whilst I was a student, oh yes, I've done my fair share of toilets, steps, supermarket floors, and corners and edges. And throughout that time, after a couple of hours of heavy labour, I remember still feeling guilty when I sat down with Dad to a normal buttered, crusty ham roll at breakfast time. It felt forbidden to give my body food. All of it – everything felt forbidden. The only way I could conceive of it being 'good' was if it was slimming bread or crackers with slimming spread and a scraping of Marmite or a dry, boiled egg. And should I ever dare to transgress, especially that early in the day, and step into the World of Forbidden Food, then I really had to go the whole hog. Should I have that little chocolate bar as well … or not? A chocolate bar for breakfast? Not a chance nowadays. Yuk, but it was deliciously bad back then, as I devoured it and sometimes went back for seconds – again, which my body didn't want, but my brain wanted.

> ▶ *All to make the most of being in the Forbidden Zone before being locked up again.*

Nowadays breakfast is a simple affair. I know what I need first thing. Often left over stir-fry from last night! Lol. When I first began Freedom Eating, it was a cup of tea (decaf or herbal when I'm in the mood, but mostly basic Tetley!), and a couple of Rich Tea biscuits. For me, back then it was heaven to just give myself permission. And afterwards, I didn't spend the rest of the day feeling like I'd started off on the 'wrong' foot, and consciously cutting down to make up for it, or ending up blowing the lot because I'd started off badly.

They say breakfast is the most important meal of the day, well, yes, for some people it can be, but hey, guess what, try drinking a big glass of water before you even begin contemplating what to eat, and see what a difference it makes to the way your head feels fifteen minutes later. My guess is, if you're anything like I used to be back then, you'll possibly even feel a little sick first thing in the morning due to being dehydrated, muggy headed, sluggish, and lethargic, your pillow feeling like a magnet. What your body's signals may be trying to tell you, and your brain is misinterpreting, is that you need water, not food or coffee. Or you may be reacting to whatever you ate yesterday, which your body didn't like.

Many diets make you feel better because they recommend upping your water intake, and it's the resulting hydration that makes you feel like it's working for you, not necessarily the strict diet regime. Or it's the clean food which most good 'diets' incorporate, which we all know is what we should be eating all the time – but we often don't. Think again if you ever catch yourself saying, 'But I feel so healthy when I'm on that diet.' Maybe your body's trying to tell you something. It may be the extra water, plus more fresh produce which is going to help your body because it's mostly water too, as well as valuable fibre. There's nothing like a good clear-out! And since a 'clear-out' needs water to help it on its way, no wonder many of us live our lives permanently constipated if we spend the day drinking nothing but diuretics like tea and coffee. At least balance it out by having extra water.

> ► *Drink as much pure water as often you can reasonably do.*

On our online support group we talk about starting the day with a hot water with a little squeeze of fresh lemon. If you really feel like a coffee, then fine, but this brings me on to another Secret

Escape Route – listen to your body and find out what's a good fit. Sometimes you can end up with a headache if you combine a coffee with a doughnut first thing in the morning, whereas if you drank the coffee, with water maybe and waited till you were sure you were genuinely hungry, body hungry, for a doughnut, then it may be perfectly okay. Or perhaps you'll need to leave the coffee till a little later in the day, or have it with two glasses of water, or black, or decaffeinated. Or change the brand, as a different one may not give you a headache at any time of day. Or never.

Certain combinations of food might not work for you. Perceived wisdom nowadays about food-combining means keep proteins away from carbs and you might be okay, less bloated and so on. But you have to do what's right for your own body. Only you know what that is.

Or maybe your body will crave tons of veggies rather than potatoes or rice or pasta. And if you can get off the sugar addiction you won't want the doughnut anyway. (See later.) In any case, many experts are saying don't have so much white bread, pasta and so on. For the odd person, though, if you insist your body feels like it, well, have it. But do wait till you're hungry enough, stop at satisfied, and make sure you observe your body afterwards. And whatever it says, at least it's not like someone else telling you what to do, it's your own flesh and blood, literally, giving you signs that something is working. Or not. And all you have to do is listen. Just listen to your body every time and you won't go far wrong.

Then, you can make the leap to complete Freedom Eating, once you allow yourself to acknowledge that luxurious fact – that no food is treasure – it's all allowed, nothing's forbidden if you practice full Freedom Eating. No food category, type or brand will ever take you out of 'safe and good' into 'bad' and the psychological Forbidden Zone again. Nothing. Ever. Again.

So you're less and less likely to fail, each time you do this. Less and less likely to end up repeating the bad patterns of the past. Once you know you *can* have it, if you're like me, you don't want it. You think about it differently. Therefore you allow yourself to consider if you actually really *do* want that flavour in your mouth right then. Maybe you won't, ever again. Maybe some days you will, some you won't. Maybe you will till your body starts to realise that this new found Freedom Eating is not just some passing fad, just like all those others have been in the past. It's for real, and it's here to stay. And you really could have cheesecake for lunch, dinner and supper if you genuinely wanted it. Body hungry, remember? But you wouldn't – not for long. That's why it works. It just ceases to be 'treasure' any more. Then you're less likely to be in 'famine' mode, and more likely to be transforming yourself into a person no longer frightened around food, scared of being let off the leash because you can't trust yourself to be 'good'. Oh my God, it's so life-changing, this whole Freedom Eating process.

I so want to give this gift to other people, and you will too – you'll want this new-found freedom for your nearest and dearest the same way I want it for mine. And do they all listen and are they all converted? Nope. Do they hell …

5. Suffering the Slings and Arrows

*You don't have to be fat
to have a food problem.*

People are always cynical, aren't they? It's normal for a socially conditioned adult in this day and age to doubt some raving loony who declares they can eat what they want from now on. They will always try to doubt you, but just wait, keep doing what you're doing, and the proof of the pudding will be in the – well, the *not* eating, and the new shape they'll gradually see appear on you, and the happiness and liberation you'll exude.

They will try to inflict their conditioning back on you – oh, expect it – like the girl at work, size eight, food-obsessed 'Jane' who said to me once when I'd started to really get to grips with Freedom Eating and lose weight, and was comfortably indulging in half a Danish pastry one lunchtime, 'Should you be eating that, with you being on the telly?'

Like my mum, who, before she got used to the idea of my Freedom Eating used to repeat the same old statements of my childhood – 'Don't eat that, you'll put all that weight you've lost back on again.' God, the temptation to let anger swell up and have a row, but guess who's already the winner here? It's not them. Just smile sweetly and carry on eating it. That'll make the point more than answering back ever would. Or say, 'When I chose to eat it, I didn't have you in mind.' Hee hee! Give it time, and they'll notice the new you. Then they'll want to know more about how you've done it, and that's the time to tell them more. *When the student is ready, and all that, and you're ready right now, or you wouldn't be reading this.* Even if you only do the first few stages, and leave the more daunting stuff till a later date, you're ready. Probably more ready than you've ever been in your life, and so fed up of being on the same old yo-yo treadmill; one that has so many rules you don't know where to begin. Well, start by just not beating yourself up and considering yourself 'bad' if you stray, especially first thing in the morning. If you're one of the legion of middle-aged, unhappily overweight women I hear from, who have all got to the end of their tether being stuck this size and feeling trapped and unable to do something that works, this is it.

So, for me, initially, in the old days before I learned about sugar addiction, my morning pick me up used to be a cup of tea and a biscuit about half an hour after I'd woken up and after drinking a big glass of water. That was my ideal. So I started doing it. But for years before that, I'd tell myself off if I started the day like that. And a telling off at the start of the day was a surefire way to end the day full of remorse, self-disgust, and self-pity, as well as having consumed far too many calories, all of which my bloody brain told my body to eat, because I'd started the day off being 'bad'. So I was in the 'bad zone' and could carry on acting that way, and feeling like shit as a result, and overeating to try to feel better. And I did feel better, the moment the next lot of food was in my mouth. But then the guilt came back, and the pattern continued. I had almighty binges, which I'll tell you more about later in the book. I've even devised a 'binge management' section, should you need a rescue plan.

Overeating, comfort eating, stress eating and just ... eating. And I could have broken it at any time by just being a witness not a judge, preventing more guilt and bad feeling from leading to more overeating. But overeat I did. All because my brain told me to. Even though, ironically, my body would have been happy with a fraction of that food.

Yet when I began Freedom Eating, from somewhere in the distant past my body remembered when it was in charge – being the one who made the decisions on what it actually needed in that instant – maybe this food, maybe that ... maybe just water, or maybe absolutely nothing. But beforehand I had some awful habits I just accepted as 'normal'. In fact, once my kids were born and I was at home looking after a toddler and a baby, I rarely ate at breakfast time, not even a biscuit, because I knew if I succumbed to something I perceived to be 'bad', and went down that route, I'd end up stuffing myself with all the wrong things by late afternoon. So I missed breakfast and starved myself thinking I was being' good'. So by the time I'd gone way past hunger and was actually starving, my poor body was craving everything in sight. Another Secret Escape Route is don't go past hungry 'enough' to being starving or you won't be able to hear your body's signals that it's reached satisfaction. The first few times you'll probably misjudge it anyway, and eat a little too much that time, or stop too early and need to eat again fifteen minutes later. Just remember the flying the plane analogy, it's off course for 90% of the time till the pilot makes a little correction then it's back on course again, and that's how learning Freedom Eating is.

> ▶ *Don't judge and don't be the critic, just observe and move on.*

I did find, however, pre-30 years old, that being busy helped to keep my 'problem' under wraps. Plus, before the big three-O, a couple of weeks 'cutting down' and I'd go back down to about 10st 5lb, no trouble. That may sound heavy to some people, but I've got a lovely photo of me at that time in some jeans I kept for posterity, the idea being one day I'd get into them again. The fateful 'one day' we all dream of. We all buy clothes especially for the occasion, which sit permanently in the back of the wardrobe unworn, labels intact. Do you?

But thanks to Freedom Eating, it's now in sight, at the end of a shorter, brighter tunnel. But what weight would you be when that 'one day' comes? Well, what *our* ideal weight is is just another whole category of 'rules' just waiting to be broken. You aren't going to be a Kate Moss or a Kate Middleton if your body doesn't naturally want to go there. Settle for being happy and content, and living a life outside the Food Prison and you won't end up caring what your weight is. It's whatever is natural for you once you start giving your body a chance to do the decision-making. That was another big 'Aha' for me, someone who was quite 'big-boned' and had almost always been heavier than others who looked the same as I did.

▶ *Remember, ignore the scales.*

Some of you may remember the dreadful days of Twiggy being the role model to all impressionable young females around the world. Well, if you were naturally shaped like a Jayne Mansfield or a Marilyn Monroe, tough. Maybe that was where your problems really started, at school or in your later, still formative years, when other people's opinions mattered so much to you it made you change your way of life and beliefs about yourself, in order to try to conform to their ideals? Think of Cliff Richard, the Perennial Peter Pan of British Pop. He was an upcoming young pop star in the early sixties when he heard a character on a new soap opera, *Coronation Street*, saying, 'That tubby Cliff Richard,' or something like that, and it affected him big-time, making him diet to lose the chubbiness. Is that what first started you on being a serial dieter because someone in their wisdom somewhere said you were fat? Or round? Or 'pleasantly plump', or some such throwaway remark, never realising how appalled you were and how it changed you – forever, in some cases.

▶ *Until now.*

Was it a parent, with their well-meaning, or sometimes not so well-meaning comments, said in the hope of connecting your behaviour because it just didn't fit in with their ideals? The never-ending family chants:

- *'Don't eat that, or your bum'll get even bigger.'*
- *'Should you be eating that with a shape like yours?'*
- *'Do you think dessert is a good idea when your holiday is coming up.'*

> – *'You'll never get into your bikini when we're away if you keep on eating bags of crisps all the time.'*

Equally dangerous, but not so obvious, are the subtle ones, the ones that we all tell ourselves are common sense, especially when dealing with children.

> – *'Don't eat those now, you won't eat your dinner.'*
> – *'Don't eat dessert before your main course.'*
> – *'Eat your greens and you'll get dessert.'*
> – *'You must clean your plate, just think of all those starving children in Africa/China/ Romania.'*
> – *'Don't leave your crusts.'*
> – *'Don't eat too many, only have one or two or you'll spoil your dinner.'*

Now these may be more acceptable to our way of thinking nowadays. After all, we're not 'good parents' if we don't control our children's diets, and teach them to eat well, are we? Hmmm, 'good parents/bad parents', now where have we heard this sort of dichotomy before? Think it through. We drum these rules into our kids as if they can't be trusted to get it right. Then hand them sweets and other rubbish that ruins their little bodies and mucks up their gut bacteria. (See later.) Well, if they start believing they shouldn't trust themselves where food's concerned, it means we're implying that they can't trust their bodies. What chance do they stand of developing natural eating, as they get older? We see it all over the Western world nowadays in childhood obesity, fat kids who've unlearned how to eat perfectly for their body's needs, and are now sadly eating for other reasons, and very often it's to please their parents. Ever been subject to this one?

> – *'Look, she's finished her plate, haven't you done well?'*
> – *'Been really good, eaten everything.'*
> – *'You've done well eating all that restaurant meal.'*

Why is overeating in a different place 'doing well'? A throwback to the days of rationing, I reckon, and a knock-on effect we could do without. So stop it, and spare your kids the next cycle. A little girl I know called Sam is like this. She's renowned for eating everything on her, and sometimes her brother's, plate. She is always on the lookout for food, like an animal on the prowl, always asking for more, always acting up if she doesn't get it, or doesn't get enough. She's not fat now and her mum is actually fairly skinny, but her mum has a big food problem.

> ►   *You don't have to be fat to have a food problem.*

How many of us hear a slim woman complain about her weight. 'You must be joking,' we think. 'You've got to be kidding. This is fat! I'd love to look like you!' But if a person feels it, then it's true for them, and it means they've got a food problem if their lives revolve around food – even size eight Jane at work, who's obsessed with her, and everyone else's, shape. Poor cow. I'd finished with the rest of that Danish with a smile on my face, probably leaving a bit and not feeling like another one for ages – giving me glee in my heart that I was free! Whilst she, as slim as she was, was very definitely still locked up, and the extent of her obsession, even having to watch other people's weight for them, probably means she'll never get out of Food Prison. And one day she'll be properly fat and forty and completely caught up in the whole yo-yo thing. Just wait till she has kids. Poor kids.

It's just a matter of upbringing, or background, or experiences in life that lead us to develop our current belief systems, and it's really heartbreaking that so many kids have parents who start interfering with how they would naturally eat so soon after learning to talk. Let's be honest here. Remember the baby bottle story? We wouldn't dream of forcing the rest of a bottle of formula down a baby's neck when it's firmly clamping its mouth shut and turning its head away. But as soon as the kid can understand us, we're forcing it to finish bigger quantities of food than it really needs, by saying, 'Eat all your dinner,' and to ignore their naturally quiet whisper of satisfaction. We're demanding that to fit in with our social conditioning, and the tribe's expectations, that they consume foods they don't necessarily feel like, right then and there, using blackmail or bribery to achieve our own goal. Or to let them just naturally graze a little instead of making them sit down to a complete meal because it suits you, and worse, to chastise them when they don't conform. They're hungry earlier than we are, but we make them wait. We insist on giving them biscuits to tide them over or to keep them quiet then wonder why they're all hyper and not hungry for dinner later at the same time we are. What's the message, for God's sake? 'Don't trust your body. Trust me. Have what I give you, not what you choose. Force-feed yourself, like my mum did me. You're wrong. I'm right.'

Like the snake from *The Jungle Book*, a parent has the hypnotic effect that starts the unlearning process at an early age. One of the biggest favours you could do a child is to let them eat when they're hungry, offer them good food to make their choices from and allow them to pick and choose at will. It's not good to make them wait for meals. If their little bodies are hungry now, they're bloody hungry now. Just because it doesn't fit in with your plans for mealtime, so what? Importantly, don't use sweets as reward and they won't become sugar addicted and hyper; don't offer snacks in between meals and make sure what they're offered for dinner is tasty and wholesome and you're enjoying it too. Why give a kid nuggets, chips and beans or a variation on that, for the fourth time that week, if you're having things like a tasty stir fry?

Surely a happy, satisfied youngster is more important than you getting your way about mealtime? Give a little, and adapt. I'm not saying let them eat whatever they want if it's sweets and no dinner forever, and I'm not saying this is the solution for every child out there. But I am saying just find a compromise to help them off this vicious spiral that may end up in them emulating you in adulthood. Would you really wish that on someone you love, if you hate how you are? Well, it's early enough to make a change right now. If I can, you can, believe me. I did that first Freedom Eating summer with my own two, aged, then, twelve and nine.

At May half-term, amazing things started to happen. When I first began to lay-off being finicky about what Lauren and Brad ate, and becoming a lot more relaxed and happy around meals, and broke the patterns I'd had when I was a kid, and didn't say a word about what or when or how to eat, yes, an incredible transformation started to take place. Just as I began leaving the food on my plate, and not coming out with so many artificial 'rules' about food, mealtimes, quantities and so on, just as I became less and less strict with my own eating, so Brad began to lose the puppy fat he'd gained so distinctly two summers before.

Bless his little heart, he'd been the top athlete in year five at the school sports, but a year later, he'd gained a little too much weight, his face was very full and round, his trousers began not to fasten. He wasn't fat, but he wasn't that naturally slim, like the boy he'd been before. Maybe it was a knock on effect from the tough time I was giving myself at that point, or from the stress our marriage had been going through, or maybe he was stressed about school, who knows. But he was beaten to the finish line by the younger boys in the year below in those key races at his final school sports that summer, when everyone else expected him to win, and my heart went out to him. But what was my family's reaction? 'That's because you've put on weight, Brad. If you hadn't eaten all those sweets and crisps this year, you would have won.' Poor little sod. Need I say more about the effect this then had? It was also then followed by a house move away from everything he knew, too. No wonder he was having a little bit of a problem getting into his new grammar school trousers. Until Freedom Eating.

▶ *My Kids Thank God for Freedom Eating.*

It's one thing when it affects your own life, but quite another when it impacts so profoundly on those so fundamentally important to you, like a son. Thank you Vikki and Shawn for giving me this freedom. I only hope it can help others in the same way, and it's so easy to do too. Needless to say, with the relaxing of my attitude, as well as being at that age where they start to sprout up, he'd slimmed right down by the end of that summer. Proud or what! It may have happened a bit naturally, anyway, but I knew I'd helped. My husband, Tony, however, came with a whole host of different rules about eating. He had slings and arrows of his own, just a different kind.

6. A Partner in Crime

The perils of contentment.

'She's content, that's why she's put on weight …' 'He's happily married, we all know what that does to a man.' Bigger dresses and beer bellies. The effect our partner can have on us is the next big strain in the unlearning process.

Seeking approval is, possibly, the biggest fundamental mistake we ever make throughout our lives. The late Wayne Dyer, my favourite motivational speaker and author, said, 'Be independent of the good – and bad – opinion of others.'[4] Sound advice. If only we could do it with those we love the most. Maybe you went through your childhood absolutely okay. I know a girl who grew up on a farm and had enough daily physical activity to counteract a grown man's calories. She was absolutely fine till she left home at seventeen and got comfortable with a man who loved his food and had a tendency to overeat. It's amazing how quickly we can start to override our bodies' natural signals. She then put on weight and shared his problems with food.

But don't forget should it happen to you, with a new partner, in the midst of all these new intentions, it's just as easy to bring yourself back to Freedom Eating again – gently and kindly. And then, once the kids come along, your own comments to them may be sorted, but perhaps it's your partner that's now being the Food Nag.

My own husband's problems had to be addressed too, as they obviously also had an impact on how our kids ate. My husband was a naturally slim person. He used to be a skinny but he's never in his life been 'fat'. He's 'one of them'. Mrs Food Problem marries a partner who hasn't got a clue about permanent overeating. He's never done it. His mum was, and still is, one of those who would serve the most delicious foods, but always in small quantities.

When I first started to eat with them, I always came away feeling secretly deprived, I suppose, because I felt the helpings hadn't been big enough. Oh, I was satisfied all right, her portions weren't always far off what it would take to make an adult satisfied, roughly a fistful of food (rough guide only) but my beliefs over-rode my body and I went off to stuff cakes and biscuits afterwards.

She also made lovely cakes for her family, and they all used to eat them and not feel so guilty that they then over ate in secret later. Sometimes, as a skinny, Tony would polish off a whole tin of little cakes, or pack of biscuits, but – and it's a big but – he would NEVER beat himself up about it, nor later go through the rest of the cupboard to eat loads more because he felt bad. He might have felt uncomfortable, and that's why he didn't do it again for a while. And, more importantly, he'd eat less later. And he didn't play the mental guilt-tennis a food prisoner plays every time they binge.

As a parent, Tony did, however, come out with the more subtle 'common sense rules' about meals and eating. These were indeed heavily drummed into him as a child, as well as a whole host of others I never had – about cutlery and elbows and talking during dinner and always leaving a little – and the list goes on. The so-called 'polite' rules about food and mealtimes, which were the legacy of his father and mother. If this works for you, then great, but we just knew we had to ease up on all the rules to make this work for our kids. And it paid off big-time.

Tony was always a Slim-Jim at school, and through his teens, and into his twenties. When we first met, and for some time afterwards, I was heavier than him. Not a bad achievement considering I'm 5′4″ and he's six foot tall. To some extent his 'don't care' food attitude helped me be less obsessed too. You do pick up other people's behaviour traits if you're around them often enough. And in my leaner years, before our troubles kicked in, I'd find it easier to say 'no' if he did too, to that extra square of chocolate, or that second slice of cheesecake. But having been an accomplished 'secret food criminal', the underlying habits were only in remission rather than gone forever. Tony would eat biscuits like there was no tomorrow sometimes, and cakes like they were going out of fashion – if they were his favourites. He always ate what he most liked – one of the key Secrets of Slim People – and then, out of nowhere, he'd be able to stop, just like that. He could almost always just say no to extra helpings, or dessert, anathema to me at the time, especially after a slap-up meal in a nice restaurant. Special occasion = become gutbucket. Enter Forbidden Zone. Abandon all vestiges of normal eating and fill body with food. Why are the 'eat all you can' menus so popular in restaurants? Because for most of us, we're a nation of food prisoners.

Now I know that you don't have to be a sheep as far as restaurants are concerned. You can be a free-thinking individual who asks for extra mayo on the side, and orders dessert to come at the same time as main course, and – shock, horror! – even eat dessert first if that's what you're most in the mood for. And then, in the spirit of stopping at satisfaction, and if you don't like waste at least keep the rest for later. And by stopping earlier on the main course, you can reserve a little bit of space in your belly so you can fit in a little something sweet, if you know you'll want it. But it's probably going to be a LITTLE bit, given you're probably not far off satisfied after eating dinner first.

It's just a matter of planning ahead. This means stop eating the main course before you reach satisfaction, knowing you'll take the remainder home. Great Secret – and one it's almost vital to get used to as it makes it easier to stop at satisfied rather than shovelling it all in your gob. Remember, you can almost always take the rest of the meal home in a 'to-go' box – most restaurants do them nowadays. Isn't it better to take it home rather than stick it down your neck at a point when your body isn't able to deal with it, and therefore has to store it and therefore make more fat? Most restaurants get asked for a takeaway box or 'doggy bag' all the time, and after you've done it a few times, you'll be used to it too. And so will the people you're with. They'll stop commenting as they see you gradually start to lose weight. One thing most people notice of a fatty is if they finish their plate or not. They'll be proud of you, and, more importantly, you'll be proud of you as you push the barriers back and face successive challenges in your mission to escape permanently from Food Prison, and leave stuff on your plate. Enlist their help if they ask you about it, and they'll possibly even feel like doing it themselves sooner than you or they would have expected.

It'll certainly at least be refreshing to have someone around them who is free of the shackles of food prison, illuminating the way to a much nicer land, a free place, where there are no restrictions from your brain about what type of food you eat. It's such a pleasure to eat with Freedom Eating, where every option is judged the natural way, the way it would have been had we never meddled with our body's control mechanisms. If you have any problem with this, it is usually all about convention. Well, buck the system! Don't kowtow to other people's ideas of what you should do, or to your partner's. It feels so fantastic to feel one-upmanship over a skinny beautiful woman, size eight Jane, for instance. Oh, I forgot to tell you, the Danish pastry episode was after I'd already let go the fact that she'd secretly put sweetener in my tea instead of the sugar I'd asked for! Buck the system. Speak up for yourself if you want to, if you can't make yourself ignore their comments with a smile. Like I did with Jane.

'Do you know,' I said, a warm fuzzy feeling pervading through me, 'this is precisely how I have been losing weight, over ten pounds now, believe it or not.' And then I smiled in a way she knew I meant it and left, knowing she couldn't quite fathom how it was possible. As I said, now *there's* a girl with major hang-ups about food. She's a chubba-lubba waiting to happen. Because with beliefs so strong she even wants other people to obey the rules *she* lives by, it'll only be a matter of time before one day the rules get the better of her, and she caves in and stuffs herself as a way of life. Over and over again, till she gets fat. She's a fat person in a skinny's body. It's a novel concept, but I believe it's true. She may look great, but she's bloody miserable, and more than that, she doesn't enjoy her food. Mealtimes are probably just as much a nightmare to her as to you and originally to me. So one day she'll burgeon.

Hate to say it, but it was far too much self-righteousness for me. I mean, fancy even secretly deciding I shouldn't have sugar in my tea! Poor girl, quite funny really. Know someone like that? Well, next time, things will be different. I promise you. Just give Freedom Eating a go, and your whole life will change. And once you start Freedom Living, you'll never want to live any other way again. For instance, have a starter as your main meal if that's the food your body is crying out for. With extra side orders if you want. Or just have a few side orders as your meal. Check in with your body and see what jumps out at you from the selection on offer, and if you're not sure, why not order both and see what then tastes the best, because that's what your body will be needing: whatever tastes the best. So eat that till you're satisfied, and take the rest home.

▷ *Break down the barriers in your life!*

Do it, in front of everyone! Especially if that dish was so delicious you'd like to repeat the experience later on at home. Why waste it once you're past satisfied and it just doesn't taste so good any more? And what's more, you are now officially totally freed from the necessity to do the opposite, and finish off other people's portions! Or 'eat it just because it's there.' Or Mum cooked it specially, or the kids left it or I haven't got a container to take it home in and it's expensive ...

They are all reasons your mind suggests to override your body's needs and requirements, but you don't have to live that way any more. Sure sometimes, something may be so delicious you just feel like eating a little too much of it. But satisfied means not being able to feel the food in your stomach even a little bit, and if you can, but it was worth it, because it was just so enjoyable, guess what, you're not going back to prison! You have been given an official perpetual 'Get Out of Jail Free' card valid for the rest of your life. So don't forget you always theoretically carry it, and can use it whenever you need to, in order to remind yourself you don't behave like that any more – and the great news is, this can apply to partners too. I don't think I've ever known The Man to be hung up on what he's eaten. On what he's drunk, maybe, but that's another story!! (And incidentally there's a nod to the need to address a drink issue too, later in the book – see the 'guise' called Della.)

What a weird unimaginable way to live your life, not being hung up on food!

I always thought it was inconceivable that someone could actually walk away from mints on the table at the end of a meal. Wasn't it part of some unwritten code that you simply have to eat them all? And also eat anyone else's left lying around? Why not just fill your home with your favourite after dinner chocolate mints and then they won't hold such a fascination if you allow yourself them on a regular basis. You won't really want many, either, if you're like me.

Christmas dinner was another big occasion for a blowout of enormous proportions. Why does everyone do it? If we did it all year round, it wouldn't have 'scarce' attached to it, and come December 25th, maybe we could reach the Queen's Speech at 3pm without feeling like our stomachs were going to explode, and being unable to do anything except sit in a corner snoring and dribbling for an hour amidst wrapping paper, toys with run-down batteries and nut shells.

And another thing, as a natural 'skinny', The Man could actually go to watch a film and not want popcorn. What? Sometimes I'd go to the pictures just to eat the popcorn! Nowadays, I rarely feel like it, and certainly don't eat it whilst watching a film. If I do buy any, and not just pinch a couple of someone else's, I'd eat it before the film, so that I followed another Secret Escape Route from Food Prison, given to me like a file in a smuggled in cake, from Vikki and Shawn.[5] Don't do anything else at the same time, so you can enjoy the food to its fullest, and not feel at the end that someone else must have sneaked up and scoffed some because you don't remember eating that much.

7. Hunger on a Plate

For food lovers everywhere – how to get the most out of your meal.

Do you know what? The best thing you can do to achieve the benefits of Freedom Eating is don't do anything else during mealtimes. This helpful hint has been one of the most instrumental in letting me understand my body. Why? Because you can hear its signals more clearly when you're not being distracted. Especially if you've made sure you're not thirsty and you're not sugar-addicted. Focussing on food is also one of the easiest things you can do as a first step. The first change to eating your way out of Food Prison gradually.

Particularly if you feel you can't let go of a diet plan or you're already going to a slimming club, this tip is worth its weight in gold. Just do the basics first, and then afterwards you can work your way up to full Freedom Eating gradually. When I started doing the Freedom Eating system, around May 1999, this was the part which took the most effort. I'd always done more than one thing at once, even down to watching the TV and reading at the same time. It used to infuriate the hell out of hubby Tony. Maybe being on constant open earpiece for my TV work made this an automatic habit, listening to what they were saying in the gallery via my earpiece, sometimes to a much more interesting conversation than you were having yourself live on air. At the start of Freedom Eating, I found it all so fulfilling and rewarding, I actually soon found myself WANTING to sit out in the kitchen and eat on my own, or on our own, instead of taking food into the lounge in front of the TV. Once Freedom Eating became our way of life, the family rarely ate in front of the telly. It helped to keep the cream coloured sofa clean too, mind you! But a by-product of this is that we were having family meals around a table together, which was great for communication and a bit of 'us' time.

> ► *Don't do anything else whilst eating – sometimes not even talking.*

Another tip for when you first begin is give yourself the permission to eat alone, just so you can savour every amazing mouthful as the Meg Ryan moment takes over. If you make similar noises as she did in the film, you may have to! And it definitely helps you know when to stop. A fistful of food, remember? That's not a huge overloaded plateful of food – even if you're out and you've paid for it.

I also used to find it a bit infuriating when Tony didn't take advantage of the Help-Yourself-Salad-Bar like all my lot did. Ah, yes, the Pizza Hut help-yourself salad bar. I remember it well. I was the expert in standing the cucumber up around the edges of the bowl to make it deeper, so I could stack the plate up higher and then eat the lot before the pizza arrived at the table. And I won't even begin to tell you about that self-service holiday at Pontins. Okay I might later. Or the as-much-as-you-can-eat Chinese meals we had. No wonder our family nearly all have a tendency to chunkiness! The embarrassment of walking back through the restaurant with a huge plateful was far outweighed by the feeling of victory in my bones as a result of greedy-pig tactics beloved by my family.

Family rules and habits are some of the hardest to break, aren't they? Being the eldest of five kids – seven in our family in total – had its advantages when it came to getting my share of treats. All. My. Childhood.

For instance the packets of cakes which came in fives. After Mum and Dad had gone shopping on Friday each week, all hell let loose. If you didn't get yours early, you wouldn't get it at all. So you ate it whether you were hungry or not! So everything basically was gone by Monday, and the rest of the week having re-activated our sugar addictions, we were all constantly on the lookout for extras. If I'd known what I know now, if someone had just told me all this then, I would have found everything so much easier to cope with. I'd have found life easier to cope with!

▶ *After all, the warning signs of gluttony were there even in the early days.*

One of my earliest memories relating to food was once I'd reached about ten. The slightly tubby young Debbie Flint was featured in a picture with the other kids from the Wandgas Cricket Club, on our first proper holiday away together, to Warner's in Hayling Island. It was fab. Left to our own devices more or less the whole week, meals at our own pace with the parents safely tucked away in bars or around the pool, and I thought I was the bee's knees in that short yellow dress. Let alone the little top and beige hot pants. But when the photos came back I saw a big round belly and made up my mind to start watching my weight – like Mummy did. So bang went my final memory of thinking of myself as slim. From then on, I classed myself as one of the fatties. I wasn't, of course. But the inevitable classroom comparisons between the cuddly, the slim and the downright skinny girls didn't help.

Later on, neither did the vicious self-consciousness of being a teenager – giving rise to an evil division between those of us who were regarded as fat, and those who were thin. The thin ones could fit into all the latest suede skirts and halter-tops from Chelsea Girl, and hot pants were par for the course. But my noticeable pudgy bits inside the tops of my thighs were the bane of my life in those pre-midi skirt days, and soon, sure enough, I began to feel guilt surrounding food.

▶ *I started to diet, at age twelve.*

Exercising all that deprivation and control was all my mind needed to tip me over the edge. No more balance. The spiral had begun. Thing is, I did manage to get a little slimmer over the course of the next two years. And by the time I left Morden Farm Middle School in Merton, SW London, I considered myself a seasoned dieter. My first grown-up clothes for high school from Martin Ford in Sutton were slimming and fashionable. But little did I expect that by the next Christmas, they wouldn't fit me. If I'd known that diets don't work, it never would have happened.

There was some element of being 'grown–up' if you had to watch what you ate, wasn't there? All the 'It' girls were on diets, weren't they? And you could easily do it, even at school, if you had the determination and drive. Back in the final year at middle school, I'd just skip lunch and sit outside getting more and more starving. We'd learned that no one realised or checked up once you were in the top year. So we starved ourselves in front of each other, but got progressively hungry as the long afternoon wore on. More than ready by the end of school to get home and immediately wolf down about four slices of marmalade on toast, in private, on my own. Then also have dinner later. I always ate it because Mum expected me to. It was completely alien to leave it. In later years I'd even have two evening meals, one at the boyfriend's and then one back at mine when he dropped me off, because we'd forgotten to tell my mum we'd eat at his house, or vice versa. Overload city. But at least I didn't get told off.

But I firmly believe having delicious school dinners with a family background like I had, was at the crux of the first true food problem I ever had, and loving food like I did, and with an inherited set of rules I had, what chance did I stand? What chance did any of us stand? I'd always loved the school dinners – ours were heaven at Morden Farm Middle School with the on-site kitchens and amazing cooks. I have never since tasted such bliss in a custard pot.

Prior to the skipping meals season, I'd regularly finish up any extras left by the skinnies on our school dinner table at lunchtime. Already my brain had forgotten how to do 'satisfied'. Already I had discovered the Forbidden Zone, and camped out there every dinner break. How much was I in my element if it was a dinner that my schoolmates and juniors on my table didn't like? And who fought hardest to be monitor on the table with the 'emaciated' first year pupils who never liked the skin on the custard? All the more for me! Oh my God, I remember being in rapture at mealtimes in those days. Thing is, unbeknown to me, those little skinnies were also in rapture, they just knew when to stop.

The Queen's Jubilee in 1977 also stands out in my mind. By now I was fifteen, and should have known better. Our street was having our party in the school hall. The night before, all the packets of cakes, biscuits and sweets were delivered to the stage, and sat lined up in row after row of stodgy indulgence, a silent witness to our great nation's need to eat crap at times of celebration. Everyone had gone home, and as my dad was the school caretaker, I sneaked back in, supposedly to find him. I crept into the darkened hall, heart pounding – a mixture of terror and anticipation that in just a few minutes, a precious stolen few of those illicit goodies would be mine. I made my way up to the stage, and surrounded by an almost tangible feeling of awe and excitement, started to search through the bags for my best choice of booty. Chocolate Snowballs or Wagon Wheels? 'Everyone's a fluffy one' marshmallow biscuits or Cadbury's Fingers. I tried to take from bags where it wouldn't be noticed, no one would have kept a record of what went where, surely? I knew there was far too much food for the party, and tried to reason with myself that it was okay, it was my right to steal away some of these forbidden fruits long before anyone else had the chance to get at them. How I thought it was my right, God only knows. But I remember the feeling of immense satisfaction when, armed with all four hot properties under my arm, I crept back home in smuggler mode.

My bedroom was the scene of a crime of the stomach. Over the next few hours, I repeatedly went back upstairs to eat 'just one last one' from the array of goodies behind the clothes in the back of my wardrobe. Narnia had nothing on me. By bedtime they were gone. The last few were forcibly eaten by telling myself that it would be best to finish the rest now, because then no one would know, no evidence at the scene of the crime. And after all – guess what – tomorrow I would be back on the diet – the one that would work this time.

I'd even have countless bad dreams about getting this unbearable panic in the pit of my stomach because I feared I wouldn't get my share of the food, doubtless linked to finding empty cake packets once too often in the kitchen because my brothers and sister got there before me.

> ▶ *Tip – in a family of six or seven, packets of five cakes isn't too clever.*

Oh, the countless bad dreams about not getting in the queue quickly enough, or being in the wrong queue, or not being able to get to the rest of the food before it was cleared away, etc etc etc. Never once do I recall feeling genuinely happy around food, or fulfilled. The shame of it is that it was all learned behaviour. 'Cos – would it really have mattered? Did my body truly want to overeat? No, it was all in my mind. What's the worst that could happen if I missed out on my share? I'd have to eat something else. Or be hungry for a little longer. God forbid we should feel hungry.

8. Hunger Know Thyself

*Three key points to help you
escape from Food Prison!*

1. Treat hunger as a friend.

*2. Don't practise prevention eating
if you're not hungry enough yet.*

*3. Learn 'pacing' to help time your
hunger right. (See later.)*

In Food Prison, we're terrified of hunger. We fear it as if it would strike us down and should we let its probing claws gnaw away at our stomachs for more than a couple of seconds, we panic. We stuff food in our mouths and once we've started, we just keep doing it. So to avoid it, we take precautions – it's called prevention eating, 'to avoid hunger in case I don't get the chance to eat later on.'

Hunger is one of the body's most basic signals that it's time for fuel. You need to feel it, and you shouldn't eat before you do feel it. This was also a Grade One Revelation for me. So don't eat before you are properly hungry, and don't carry on eating after you're *satisfied*. Hunger shouts, remember, so you will definitely know you're hungry. Other signs apart from distinct pangs include:

- Feeling slightly giddy.
- Feeling a little sick.
- Feeling a little panicky.
- Feeling that you can't concentrate.

There are medical reasons for each of these alternative signs of being hungry – google it, and the functions of hormones 'leptin' and 'grehlin'. All you need to do is experiment a little. Wait. Observe. Note it for next time. Play the scientist. Conduct your own observational tests to see which sign means what for you. Think, 'What's my body trying to tell me here?'

This is a biggie – it could just be, 'I'm thirsty.' If we are, it's possibly the reason for many of the signals our body gives out during the day, since many of us are so dehydrated the chemical and electrical reactions in our bodies just can't work properly. So they send out distress signals, which manifest themselves as a multitude of different symptoms. Including hunger.

Best treatment? If you're not distinctly hungry, but you don't know what you want, and something isn't quite right and you feel you need to take some action – then just drink a big glass of water. Sounds simplistic, but you'll soon know if it was hunger, because it'll be back again in fifteen minutes or so. At which point you could eat some food, but listen to your body's next signal and only choose what it's really crying out for – what your body wants, not what your mind thinks your body wants. Imagine the food in your mouth. Smell it. Even taste a tiny bit if needs be. Imagine it in your stomach having eaten it. Does it feel right? Then try it. Don't do anything else at the same time, just sit and savour every mouthful. Don't get the next one ready till you've swallowed the first. Give your body's hormones a chance to start reacting to the food being eaten rather than wolfing it down before your body's even noticed it's coming. Then you're more likely to notice 'satisfied'. Eating was designed to be pleasurable, like sex, also necessary for the survival of the species, so it's no accident these vital 'tasks' feel so good. Then monitor what's happening to your body and stop when the taste of the food suddenly isn't 'blow your mind fantastic' or Meg Ryan any more. It can still taste good, but not incredible, so stop. Yes, I said stop! Especially when you start noticing your own most distinctive signs.

How to know you are 'satisfied'

You may take a deep breath. You may start being distracted by what's going on around you. When you haven't yet eaten enough, eating will be the only thing on your mind, believe me. When your mind starts wandering off onto other topics, you're probably satisfied. You'll have waited, of course, till you were hungry in the first place, and the rewards of the resulting heightened pleasure for the taste buds, near ecstasy sometimes, will be yours for the taking. Freedom Eating brings with it the most wonderful eating experiences. You're not feeling deprived, possibly for the first time in your adult life. You're choosing what your body wants most and what tastes best, each and every time. You can, if you choose (that is if it's what your body wants) have anything because nothing is forbidden. You're not eating things just for the sake of it, or because you feel you have to, or because it's still sitting there looking at you, or because you've always reached out automatically and said 'yes' without thinking, because you've been so used to saying 'yes' if it meant allowing yourself a little unexpected treat. Emotional eating will be no more. This is a biggie as I was to find out in later months. Forbidden territory will be no more, and you are having the unique experience, almost certainly for the first time you can remember, of stopping eating when you still feel comfortable.

▶ *Stop when you're satisfied.*

Maybe even leave a little on your plate. Yippee it's possible! That's Freedom Eating in a nutshell, and if you want to try it out, then start right away. See if you can do it at the next mealtime. Take a few baby steps towards a giant leap of faith that will set you free of food prison forever. And you can start by waiting till you're really hungry the next time you eat. See the later guidelines, some specifically for people who choose at this stage to combine it with existing diet plans, and get stuck in. And keep re-reading this book or checking out my website for new information, as it's essential to reinforce the new behaviour.[6]

▶   *You'll never change a lifetime's bad habits by reading just once.*

– *It's deciding to do it.*
– *It's taking action to make it happen.*
– *Then reinforcing that new behaviour again and again.*
– *Plus relying on the Support System Treats to help you find other coping mechanisms and to make the changes permanent.*

▶   *Just remember that those closest to you may find it all a little perplexing.*

9. What 'They' Say

Even your children can break free
from the pattern if you do it first.

More slings and arrows, I'm afraid.

You might change you, but you won't change them as readily, especially not overnight, unless they're really open-minded, or desperate to change. So just accept that some people in your life will just have to learn later than others, and only tell them in detail when you feel the time is right, when they start asking about your new outlook, or your new shape. So many people live their lives based on other people's opinions. I did as well, to be honest. Others' opinions were the most important thing in my decision making process. So if I heard too loud and too clear that others thought I was wrong, I'd just give up. Why do you think we took on board all these erroneous rules about eating in the first place? We must have believed their perpetrators to be right, or we would have ignored their comments and 'advice'. But thing is, a lot of our habits stem from having our beliefs overruled from a young age.

▶ *I can never say all this enough. Think about it.*

– *'Don't trust your body to get it right, trust me.'*
– *'Mummy knows best.'*
– *'Why do you want to eat that now, put it back?'*
– *'You're in my house and you will do as I say.'*
– *'Why? Because I said so.'* Oh dear, oh dear, oh dear.

Don't feel too bad if you recognise yourself in any of this, I was a 'worst offender' because I was just doing what my mum and peers and siblings had done to me. And so the cycle continues.

> ▶ *Unless you break the cycle by becoming aware*
> *right now.*

It'll be the best gift you could ever give someone, especially a child. To not have them 'unlearn' their body's perfect eating signals. Wow, what a thought. Do you recall any memories of weird behaviour around food? Linked to deprivation and control? Why would a new human being, born with a perfect eating mechanism completely override their body and its signals, to participate in such bizarre food rituals? Why do we do it to ourselves? Why do we do it to our children? My mum, bless her, is a chief offender. She does it as a matter of course, quite naturally, when confronted with the enemy – food. And just like many chief offenders, she vehemently denies it. I recall once commenting to her about a book we'd interviewed someone about on 'Live at Three' with Jayne Irving on Living in 1997. It was basically saying that you're the results of your mum's eating habits – if she dieted, then you, as her daughter, will almost certainly repeat the sins of the mother in your adult life. It makes sense. You see it happen, assume that's how things are done, and fall naturally into that pattern when your time comes. Say the same things, make the same observations, feel the same guilt, lose a few pounds, gain a lot, lose a few, gain a lot, and end up looking just like her eventually. Words of wisdom from a mother's lips are taken as gospel, especially when you're too young to know better, subconsciously shaping our ritual beliefs and determining our food destiny.

So I told Mum about this book and its claim. 'I haven't got a food problem,' she indignantly replied. 'I could tell you everything I've eaten for the last two days.' That's my mum, indignant. 'I know what to do, I know what I should and shouldn't eat,' she declares, merrily delving into my fridge as soon as she walks in through the door. Mostly cuddly or voluptuous through the years, and sometimes really big and buxom, my lovely old Dad loved every bit of her, 'his bit of meat'. But at her largest she seemed very unhappy. She'd eaten her way there through five children and a complete lack of understanding of portion sizes, and now fashion dictated she should be slim. So she basically joined the yo-yo brigade from there on in. She did get really thin one year. She and my sister did – with Weight Watchers. Oh, if only we could wave wands overnight – wouldn't things be different? For a time she wished she'd stayed there at that skinny weight, looking slightly emaciated with no bust to speak of, but fitting into skinnies' clothes and feeling good when she looked in the mirror, and feeling crap when she looked in the fridge.

Vikki Hansen was a slimming club instructor and has grave doubts about the long-term losses sustained by club members. According to findings, over 90% of the people put it right back on again. So they really are still food prisoners when they have lost the weight, left the class and gone back to being 'normal'.[7] So many of us know people like that. Or we are people like that.

Isn't it true? The phrase, 'I really must go back to slimming club,' in one form or another, has been heard time and time again through the years. The same people. The same problem back again, the same ten or twenty pounds to lose.[8]

▶ *Break the pattern. Break out of that food prison.*

Get Freedom Eating and you will stay out, permanently. It's so easy. Really. So many people can testify to how permanent this system is. And do you know why? Why it's so logical and it works? Because it's eating the way nature intended. Eating the way you were born to. Kids, young kids, left to choose their own food from a selection, chose a balanced diet over the course of the week. After the first few days of eating all the junk – and that's only because they've already been subject to some form of deprivation and control – they then actually chose to eat the veggies as well as the meat, the fruit as well as the pies, and sometimes they only ate the fruit, or the salad, or the broccoli. Dare you try it with your own kids? I tell you what, it's really liberating to not have to stand guard at the door of their stomachs and to not have to chastise or goad or bribe or threaten your way through mealtimes. Give it a go, and you'll set them on the path to freedom for the rest of their lives too. If you still don't see the value of this to yourself, if, for instance, you've been trying it for a few weeks and haven't quite got the hang of 'satisfied' yet, don't give up, your family need you to stop your vicious food cycle, they need you to be happy, don't they? You owe it to them, and yourself, to keep trying. Just persevere.

And stop beating yourself up about it all. Relax. Get calm. See it through. Work out what's been missing, adjust, and step right on up to the next level. The pace of change is completely individual. Some people can notice big differences quite quickly whereas others sometimes put on a little before it starts to come off, gradually getting the hang of the eating the Freedom way, and becoming a totally different person around food. And hearing others' experiences and seeing yourself in them makes you realise you're not alone in all this. (See later for the six different 'guises' of Freedom Eater.)

My experience of slimming clubs

I'm someone who hates being told what I can't do as it just makes me want to do it more. The very thought of going to a club I'm not looking forward to attending anyway, where there's a chance someone could be telling me I've been 'bad' this last week, and scrawling in a little unhappy face into my record book, then sitting talking about the very thing we're trying to make less important in our lives in order to become 'normal' – food – and what we are allowed, and what foods are 'sins'. Well, God knows why I even bothered going to my first club back in the Dark Days of Screensport in Cheshire. Desperation, I suppose. I'd got to the stage where I was eating food from the bin, that spag bol I described earlier on. I'd gone to get slimming pills. I'd come off the pill to lose that quarter of a stone it had put on me a couple of years earlier. I'd done the gym thing. I'd tried the F-plan (and we all know what happened with that one! Instead, see the 'Debbie-F (that's me!) Plan' later). And nothing worked. This was also the time that Mum and Linda, my sister, had done so well. They were skinny, I was really, really heavy, and self-conscious about it too, and they nagged me.

'It's worked for us,' they cried, unable to see why their way was not going to work for me. Linda had just become a slimming club instructor herself, her great big fat picture from a few years earlier sat in my bedroom looking at me every time I came back for a visit to Mum's. So off I went. It was a local club in Northwich, and pleasing to my eye when I walked in the door and saw loads and loads of people far fatter than me. But they were the ones smiling when in week three, I'd actually gained back the two pounds I'd lost the week before, plus an extra one into the bargain. Must have been someone else's fat, is all I can say! And the chat wasn't great either, just obvious stuff I really did know. And there lies the problem. There must be few serial dieters who don't know most of what we should do. The problem is getting yourself to do it consistently. As Anthony Robbins says, keep saying, 'I should do this, I should do that,' and pretty soon you'll 'should' all over yourself.[9] (Say it fast ... get it?!)

'I should' belongs on 'I'll try' street. You can make the decision in an instant, for instance to give up smoking. It's the sticking to it afterwards that can be the problem. The 'challenge', should we say?

▶ *And that's where Freedom Eating really comes into its own.*

Because what you're looking at is adopting a whole new thought process, a whole new way of eating and a whole new permanent system to help you break free and get liberated. And stay there. Once you start doing it, the weight coming off is the side effect of adopting a new, healthy approach to food and mealtimes, rather than the primary aim. What you end up doing is actually the very thing you'd started overriding all those years ago.

> ► *That's why this system is so different from any other.*

My research into what was around back then included a couple of different obscure audiobook sets from the States. Very intense they were, too. They had a few things in common with some of the ones I researched from the UK, mainly the visualisation techniques and affirmations, and I believe there's a lot to be said for all that. After all, it's definitely true that what you focus on expands, so if you say you're going to lose weight, but inside you actually believe you're a fat person, you'll almost certainly break the diet at the first hurdle. It's going to take a lot of mind conditioning to shake free the deep down opinion that you're useless, you 'always' eat too much, you 'never' lose weight no matter what you do. But it's possible. We all know that, unless you have a medical condition, the only way you get fat and stay fat is by eating more food than you use up in energy on a consistent basis. The only way you will lose weight and keep it off is by eating less than you have been, as well as preferably, exercising more, and now Freedom Eating to keep it off for good. We all know that, so why don't we do it? Well, perhaps by dieting consistently we've interfered with our own bodies. A traditional diet of deprivation and control leads to a lowered metabolism as your body gets starving regularly and trips into famine mode, yo-yo dieting through the years will never work long-term, and will lead to stress galore.

If you're one of those people, and hate diets and they never work, then you will be able to forget the diets forever if you learn Freedom Eating. Or you may use it alongside any traditional diet – any. Either way, you'll gradually go back to trusting your body to guide you in choosing what, when and how much to eat. But how did we get here in the first place? Was your life like mine?

10. More from the Fat Lady

The biography continued -
Bridget Jones eat your heart out.

I'll never forget my first encounters with Freedom Eating. I've already mentioned it in the preface, but here it is in a bit more detail, just to see if my experience resonates with you. Especially at this point, as by now you might have dabbled a bit with trying the methods I've been discussing so far, and it'll be nice to compare notes.

The turnaround happened in the spring of 1999. A couple of eureka moments tied in with the arrival of the authors of *The Seven Secrets of Slim People* from America and an insight I'll never forget. My job at QVC the Shopping Channel – source of stress and so much of the weight gain over the past five years – was now to be the source of my salvation. Shawn Goodman and Vikki Hansen, appeared on air with their book and (then cassette) tape pack, telling us all about the way they now lived their lives without worrying about weight gain, or food, or calories. The system was called Freedom Eating.

Ha ha ha, funny joke – you're free to eat what you want, that's right, isn't it? That's what everyone says, and it's true. But the crucial difference here is the 'want' bit. I read the book with interest. *The Seven Secrets of Slim People* ... hmmm.

▶ *Eat till you're satisfied, not till you're full?*

I did the show immediately after their first appearance, and spoke about this on air. 'What,' said Mrs Thirteen Stone, 'you mean you don't keep eating till you can't breathe any more?' Ha ha, funny fat lady. Again.

But the book had me hooked, and I really and truly started

to see a way out of the eternal food prison in which I'd made my HQ and set up permanent camp. That summer, until their next visit, and my first show with them, I devoured the book and it clicked – so I semi-practised these new alien principles. You know how you always think it's your little secret – people don't realise how bad this food thing really is for you? You have to deal with it alone, or in secret, or you're a failure? Well, surprise, surprise, you're not alone. And neither was I, it transpired, as page after page made me realise just how common this issue is. Keep reading this book, and if you're just like me, it might click with you too. After twenty long years of 'having a food problem', at last I was finding out the secrets of slim people. And the good news is – we can be like them. Keep a diary, like I did, to chart your progress.

After a slightly shaky start, once I'd let go of the old behaviours that were sneaking back in after the 'half a pound slimming club experience', I soon found the weight started dropping off me. It's funny because it's so long ago now, that I am delighted when I hear from others who remind me just how much of a revelation this system was at the time for me. A lovely make-up lady called R recently became very interested in my book when I told her I was doing a revision, and two weeks later she reported back to me that she'd lost half a stone without even trying. Well, my first month or so led me to be nine and a half pounds lighter. Easily. I was amazed!

It all actually seemed to be working – you really can have the best of both worlds – be 'normal' around food and eat what you like, and have a great shape. Well, I was moving in the right direction. Two inches off my waist at that stage! It was doing my morale, and my sex life, the world of good. I was starting to see my ribs again. I used that old chestnut, the visual equivalent in pats of lard, on a big tray, to show how much fat I'd lost from my body and it rammed the point home. Do it too – then losing 'only a pound or two' won't feel quite so tiny – assuming you can't give up the scales. My pile of lard was growing and growing, only now

I was carrying it on a tray onto my shows and not on me, and I felt like a new woman.

I really can't overestimate how amazing that feeling was, to finally feel like someone had waved a magic wand because the system was working so well for me. I just 'got it,' and according to my online support groups, many others do too.

Now, the insights I had been collecting over the first six months started to be very useful as I recounted my experiences to others who began noticing this massive change in me. The first insight was illuminating – it was around the time I first saw the two ladies with their system on QVC.

Back home, I'd had marriage problems the year before, and we'd come through them. Or so I thought. At the heart of my problem was the reasoning, 'If only I was slim then he'd want me more and there wouldn't be a problem. If I was able to eat normally and not have a food problem then so many things in my life would be okay.' Familiar one, huh? Well, me and The Man were in the kitchen and I was, as usual, sounding off about weight and food and blah blah blah. And he chirps up: 'But you eat quite normally, don't you? It's not like you're always eating rubbish, you eat quite healthily really, don't you?' Stunned silence. Me and the 'N' word in the same sentence, in the same sentence as eating habits. *Normal?*

I thought about it long and hard. Well, actually, yes, I did usually eat healthily. I didn't stuff myself every night. You know the amazing before and after pictures in the paper about slimmers of the year who have shed ten stone and they got there in the first place by gorging on chips and curries and beer and chocolate. That was never me. But I thought of myself in the same terms, as they did, no doubt.

- *'Jerry Springer, I have a food problem.'*
- *'I see. Well, pardon me for saying it, but, Debbie, you don't even look big and fat.'*
- *'But I am fat, Jerry. I feel fat. I've been bad.'*

- '*Well, let's see how you feel when we bring on Angela. Angela – come on out here. You see, Angela's over twenty stone – 280lb – now look at **her** and say you've got a problem ... a problem, a problem, a problem ...*'

Like a dream sequence, it all unfolded in my mind. And I asked myself some basic questions. How can I possibly class myself as having a problem, when I'm nowhere near as bad as others? Can't explain that one, so what do we do? We just put up, shut up, and eat up, always in solitude, always in guilt city, but invariably with supreme satisfaction when the food is in our mouths and going down bit by precious bit.

▶ *This technique set me free. Full stop. Period. End of story.*

You just have to follow the guidelines, and find some faith in your own body that *it knows what to choose*, and how much to opt for, and when to stop. Never again reprimand or lecture yourself, or class whole categories of food as off bounds. Trust your body. So I did.

It had been working so far. But it was still early days, and there was actually no reason to think that my gradual weight loss would stop as long as I was listening to my body and eating the way nature intended. And on it would go until my body reached its ideal weight. Its own natural weight, which may not be the weight which I'd choose, but this way at least I get to break free from food prison for the rest of my life. And it's a nice place to be.

Because I've changed my eating habits – easy bit. Since discovering Freedom Eating all those years ago there's been no bingeing. And I'm mainly sticking to it – hard bit. But I'm not on a diet, or counting, or beating myself up – good bit. I'm getting guidance from a proven, reliable system – easy bit. And I'm putting it into action – challenging bit. If it's that easy why is it challenging? Because of the habits of a lifetime and because we are all human – with an Inner Chimp built in.

We know what we should do. Knowing's the easy bit, right? And it always has been, it's doing it that's the problem. But this time, I thought to myself as I looked in the mirror at a body pushing towards a stone lighter, one big thing was different. I wasn't having the eternal torture of sabotaging myself at the slightest provocation. You know the form – 'I've eaten one biscuit too many so I'll blow the diet, eat the lot and start again tomorrow.'

Sound familiar? How many 'last suppers' have you had in your time? Once newcomers to Freedom Eating finally get it, and the penny drops they tell me things like this:

> *I'm calmer, more full of conviction that I know this time is different, this time I'll do it. Instead of beating myself up about it every time I stray off the track or make the slightest mistake. I'm happily going through the most massive change my body has experienced since I initially learned to over eat when I was a child.*

This is the process of changing every habit to do with food, mealtimes and eating – it's life-changing. And back then, boy did I have a lot of changing to do.

▶ *Changing the habits of a lifetime*

In 1974, the girls in 2H who brought an apple in for break time didn't mind giving me the rest when they'd had enough after only eating half. Why leave any? My apple cores were always nibbled to the bone. My lovely old dad used to give his five kids a few slices of apple each as a treat in a bowl, and some orange segments. So to have a whole one was nowhere near as readily available as it is today. At school, the dinners were bliss and heaven: caramel tart, Manchester tart, the best custard on the planet, never yet equalled, subject of many a bad dream about being hard-done-by or not getting there in time for the sitting and having severe angst from not getting my share – those types of recurring dream. All my life I had those. Till Freedom Eating. Morden Farm Middle School in Merton, South London did after all, have a canteen second to none and it had a lot to answer for!

I wouldn't mind, but I wasn't actually fat. In fact, I was one of the slimmer ones in the family for a long time. I remember Dad giving me jip one night over how far my collar bones were protruding, and I recall feeling proud that for once in my life someone was using the 's' word on me! Skinny? No way! Only the stick insects in the class, who looked like their legs would break if you so much as looked at them on the hockey pitch, were usually associated with the 's' word. Oh, how I dreamed of being skinny.

When I was nine I drew pictures of myself, imagining what I'd be like at age thirteen, how I thought I'd have changed by then: skinny, with boobs and a boyfriend called Michael (for some reason). None of which turned out to be true. I ended up four years later, a slightly taller version of how I was at nine. With a little bit more podge round the middle – fat made solely of marmalade on toast which I'd been eating four slices of every night after school by then. And the boyfriend was not called Michael, he was called Neil Develin. Then Robert D, then Robert E, then Rob Squires. Maybe boys called Robert were attracted to chubby kids with a penchant for marmalade, I don't know.

Why is it that all my memories of school trips seem to be punctuated with mealtimes? The delicious confiture, croissants, and café au lait from Dravail, just outside Paris, where we all went for the French school trip aged eleven or twelve. Then there was all the spaghetti and my first Martini and lemonade ever in Andalo, Italy, whilst skiing at age fourteen. The theatre trip with the girls up town to see Tom Conti in *Whose Life is it Anyway?* at sixteen, which couldn't take place until I'd stopped the taxi on the way to buy up the sweet shop to eat during the show. And, of course, the *piece de resistance*, close encounters of the Pontins' self-service kind – the holiday camp never knew what hit it the year they brought in their short-lived 'help yourself' food section and my family rocked up and helped themselves to some of every option on the menu – every mealtime. When we got home we were all half a stone heavier, but wasn't that to be expected on holiday though?

There were countless other memories too, of course. But why did our family have an obsession with food? Well, the obvious reply was because there were seven of us. Being in a big family is often cited now as a big starting gun for developing 'eat it now' bad habits. I was the eldest of five, after all, and Mum and Dad went shopping on a Friday, the day after Dad got paid for his caretaker's work. This was the thing, if you didn't eat the treats there and then, irrespective of whether you were hungry or not, you would miss out. It gave it some kind of treasure status, made it elusive and sought after. And we all became very skilled at overriding our appetites and our body's signals, to allow our brain to take charge with the overriding edict: eat it now or you go without. So by Monday, all the best stuff was gone – guaranteed.

- *'Here, have another packet of crisps – there are only two packs left to go around three people.' And our body said okay.*
- *'I say, body, there are two more courses after this, are you sure you don't mind me getting another piece of garlic bread with your appetiser?' And our body said, 'I don't think so, but you're in charge, brain, you're the boss.'*

Sound familiar? And so it happens that we all *stop* listening to our bodies and do what we think instead of pausing for a minute and considering doing what our bodies *feel* like. Listening to our own needs. God forbid we should ever take any notice of our body's suggestions that we don't really want any more food just yet. Don't be so stupid, just open your mouth and *eat*. Speak now, or forever hold your piece ... of cake.

But the worst times were still to come. Still really finding my feet in the fatty stakes and, on the whole, not doing too badly at fifteen, I'd got down to an all-time low of nine stone following an apple a day diet, at lunchtime, and a child size portion of dinner at night. Or an egg and a fish finger for lunch, taken to school in a Tupperware container. In bed by 9p.m., stomach growling. Or cursing myself if I'd succumbed to temptation and committed the heinous crime of giving in to a bowl of – shock, horror – cornflakes. Every carefully counted calorie imprinted on my memory, or recorded in my five-year diary, Bridget Jones style. So I did, in fact, briefly manage to achieve a really flat stomach, and for a few short months, felt like I was truly one of the Slim People. In the mirror I was, but in the brain I was still the troubled fattie who could never be normal around food. I was fifteen, and being slim lasted two years.

At fourteen, it had been even worse. And it was really the start of the problem being a major 'thing'. I'd been in with a bunch of girls who all had similar hang-ups. I'd pigged out that summer, and had a horrendous photo taken of me with the rest of the mostly slim and nubile Merton Borough hockey team on our week-long tour to Holland. I even remember sneaking downstairs in the middle of the night to pinch a few Quality Street from a big tin kept by our unsuspecting host family. No one ever knew but me. And boy was I thrilled at my booty, three toffees and my favourite purple wrapped caramel one with the nut in the middle. If only they knew. So I had to do something about it, hence the egg and fish finger deprivation nightmare. So the next spring, Apeldoorn in Holland never knew what hit it when I returned a stone lighter, a tornado on the hockey pitch, and off the pitch, raring to get off with whomever I could in the boys team. A subsequent memory involved kissing each of the boys in turn on the coach on the way home and feeling terribly guilty when Dad found out – guilt in those days equalled several packets of Rancheros crisps and two Twixes, I seem to remember.

Anyway, after a couple of years being still pretty trim due to all the sport, despite being totally diet obsessed, I began driving my boyfriend mad with ceaseless 'Does my bum look big in this?' inquisitions. Veering between being 'good' and being 'bad', by celebrating every birthday or anniversary, or family business getting its first bank loan, with a meal out. A big meal. Mostly with my first long-term, official, grown-up working boyfriend, Martin, aged eighteen. And mostly at The Safari Steak House in Lower Morden.

So here we were, I remember it so well. Prawn cocktail, then fillet steak, buttery jacket potato, peas and onion rings. Bread and butter. Diet bitter lemon (got to make some effort, huh), and their speciality dessert, the gut-busting banana split, covered with cream and ice cream and canned fruit cocktail pieces to follow. Then coffee with lots of cream and sugar, mints, and, on this occasion, even a little cheese and biscuits forced down my neck. Then, after all that food, way more than my body needed, the thing my body wanted most was … a sick bag. As far as drinking was concerned, I was never one for a drink, but Martin polished off a couple of lagers on top of all that. But then Martin was naturally slim, and had actually left some of his other courses, some of which was also polished off by me. We stood, painfully. We walked out into the night air, slowly. And then it hit me. I was so stuffed I had to walk up and down a bit outside before I could actually bend down enough, without throwing up, to get in the car for the journey home. At least ten minutes of the walking before I could trust myself to face the five-minute car journey back to my house without turning into a scene out of the movie *Car Wash*. (The kid honked up in the car, if you don't remember!)

So there was the pattern. Reinforcement came thick and fast from my similarly obsessed family, that this was the way things should be, so that every flipping time an occasion arose, my brain took over and over-rode my body's signals like a woman possessed. 'The famine has ended! The famine has ended!' went the cry, and my mind ran around like the proverbial blue-arsed fly, acting accordingly. I probably ate enough calories on those occasions to last me three days. Then go back to being 'normal' or 'good' which equated to being on a diet, starving, or 'bad' which equated to not following a diet, 'breaking it' and starting again tomorrow – every tomorrow. But back then my 'bad' wasn't particularly bad.

In fact, I was eating 'normally,' no huge binges at that stage, but did not realise it at all and just kept punishing myself in the extreme if I strayed from the strict rules I'd laid down for my 'musts' surrounding my eating patterns. Severe Rules are another big no-no for successful weight loss. You must have suspected by now that the key to Freedom Eating is … Freedom. Freedom to unlearn all the bad things, all the unnatural things, which you've adopted as normal behaviour around food through the years.

▶   *Control and deprivation don't work – long term.*

Endless charts of unrealistic weight losses went on the wall. And soon got taken off again when there was no more room to keep changing all the dates on it, as each successive deadline came and went to no avail.

One of the only other times I ever really got slim after I left school was when I was on Larry Grayson's Easter *Generation Game* on TV in 1981. I reached a lovely 9st 10lb, about four stone less than my heaviest but I was totally one hundred per cent screwed up about it. 'Does my bum look big in this?' wasn't the half of it. Poor boyfriend, Martin, endured endless paranoia and demands for comparisons with other girls' body parts. He was having to contend with a slim girlfriend, with a fat mind. I was an undergraduate student/trainee accountant during the uni hols. I spent all day bored silly, crunching numbers, looking forward to a lunchtime Caramac chocolate bar, eaten slowly and savoured religiously and the daily call to Martin's office for a catch up, from the phone box near the YMCA in Wimbledon, naturally – mobiles were still nearly twenty years away. In the afternoon, bouts of daydreaming was interspersed with frenzied bouts of bookkeeping to make up for the lost time. I'd spent hours planning the rosy future I was creating for myself, but in all of it I HAD to be slim, as my dreams of being on TV beckoned. So did another boyfriend, eventually. Mark had a penchant for muesli and also scrambled eggs on doorstep toast, and a mum who made amazing cakes. But I was working my way through university at the time by cleaning loos and keeping Sainsbury's spic and span for Dad's new contract cleaning business and all that hard graft helped keep the weight off, to an extent. But all that extra physical work gave me a new license to consume.

If only I'd have learned then what I know now. If only someone had sat me down and explained what I found out when I discovered Freedom Eating. The logic. The liberation. The laid back lunches.

By the summer of 1983, I'd scraped through university – too many distractions in the form of theatre, an attempt at modelling, singing, and, of course, the boyfriends. I got a 2-2 and I was a BSc. Econ. Hons from the London School of Economics. Proud, and jobless. Time to knuckle down. I managed to fit into two small suits bought for all those job interviews I was going to get, but no interviews came, it was all too competitive in my obvious career of accounts. And as I turned my attention to other options, I had a rude awakening. Too late I realised I wasn't going to get any of the high–flying positions I wanted in advertising or at the BBC as a producer, without having been something extraordinary – like the Chief Editor of the London Student Magazine, or the creator of an award winning university drama transferred to the Edinburgh Festival, or having won an award like Top Student 1983. It was very competitive back then. I'd only managed to reach Co-Features Editor and to play Hortense in the LSE production of *The Boyfriend*, which someone else had produced. And even then my legs were too fat. Why *were* all the other girls' legs always so much slimmer? I swapped Hortense's miniskirted French maid's outfit for an unpopular longer version but at least in a line up with the 'skinnies' on the stage I was not the odd one out with thunder-thighs. Now I look back and wish I could wave a wand and have stayed the shape I was then. If only the control and deprivation hadn't set in in the next few years and taken my weight swings to an even greater level.

Before I left university, partly due to being happy with said boyfriends, I managed to diet and Slendertone my way into a couple of Miss Pontins finals competitions, and was quite proud of the fact I'd got there, even though standing next to the other tiny beauty queens, I knew I had no chance. Scored a couple of Twix and Rolo sessions for that one, I can tell you! But there were still no job interviews, and a life of cross casting and balance sheets (accounts terms) spread out before me, unless I did something. And boyfriend Mark was on the way out by then too, so I had to get my act together. So I sold my motorbike and paid for a three month 'How to be a radio presenter' course at the National Broadcasting School in Soho, London.

Still living at home, I totally immersed myself in this new world. I had lots of barriers to overcome, being female, having no idea about technical stuff, and having a strong south London accent, but it meant not a spare second to even consider food. Before too long I was doing all the hours that God sends, practising after-hours in their purpose-built studios, surviving on the odd yoghurt and packet of chips from the kebab shop on the corner of Greek Street, or – once in a blue moon – a Topic bar. Every night I used to come home late from Morden tube station, exhilarated, exhausted, and excited about the next day's experiences, my head in the clouds dreaming of becoming a 'proper' presenter with a 'proper' job. Oh, and of a fellow student called Andy. The weight fell off – I was busy and happy.

By Christmas, the course was over and we were all unleashed onto the unsuspecting radio community (only two or three students getting or already having jobs) the rest of us going back to what we'd done before, all the while perfecting our radio show-reels and sending off applications all over the country. But most programme controllers didn't relate to my 'silly accent' as one boss in Hull called it ... Rejection time. Despite my winning their 'Student with Most Progress' Award, yes it was rejection time – big time. Over and over. Oh, and Andy didn't love me. I forgave him years later when it turned out he was gay – but that didn't help me at the time. At the time, it just felt like another layer of rejection, heartache and several song writing sessions. And at the exact same period, one thing kicked in, bringing with it deeply ingrained habits galore – euphoria – it was Christmas!

The annual food fest – that festive, fabulous time of year when food abounds, just laid out asking to be eaten to excess, the perfect antidote to all that rejection. Lots of rejection meant lots of comfort eating that's for sure. Often in secret. That Christmas the weight piled on, and I decided to copy my kid sister Linda and went blonde. By the January, at a reunion evening out, one of my fellow students didn't recognise me from behind with most of my extra stone having gone on my bum. It was so sad. I was so sad. So I went blonder, tried to get some dress sense, went back to the accountants, and spent the next five months tearing my heart out over Andy, who saw me regularly but at arm's length ... most of the time – turns out he was still experimenting, not that he or I knew that back then. I wrote reams and reams of soul-searching, heartstring-pulling prose about my feelings for him, none of which worked, apart from to make me feel better temporarily by getting it all out, and to set up a pattern that was to repeat itself on a regular basis for the next couple of decades of my life, packed with journaling. I cross-cast neat columns of numbers on an adding-machine by day, dreamed of Andy all night, and ate chocolate, biscuits and pizzas throughout the entire period to lighten the load. And put on even more weight.

Then I discovered diet pills. By mid May 1984, I was winging my way to Corfu for my first ever foreign holiday with my (slim) mate, Gill, and her (slim) sister and her sister's (skinny) friend. By late May 1984, I was winging my way back again, half a stone heavier – a neat achievement in two weeks considering my determination not to – and about to start a whole new era for myself working for a fledgling sports cable TV company called Screensport in Knutsford, Cheshire. The big move, leaving home at last. Thinking back, I now remember something strange – my family had gone on holiday during my 21st birthday, and were still away when I packed up my little world into my Ford Fiesta and left home. Hmmm – back to the whole theme of making others think I was okay and others all assuming I could go off on my own and just get on with things. I'd never do that to one of my kids now, but of course a big family of five meant I was kind of just left to my own devices, which had both benefits and disadvantages. I just never realised how the disadvantages played out subconsciously in a blanket of food.

Auntie Peggy offered me a room for a couple of months, and I gratefully took up her offer, finding, to my delight, that I was able to successfully challenge myself to eat all her saved up Christmas goodies –Peggy was tiny and a chain-smoking natural skinny. Boxes of chocs still under the telly. 'Help yourself,' she said. So I did. And so it went on, including the new-found delight of Manchester bakeries' delicacy, vanilla slices. Just how much weight could I put on? Eleven and a half stone was easy. Nudging eleven and three quarters, bulimia finally came knocking on my door. Soon after, and left to my own devices, I sought solitude in the form of my very own first house in Wincham near Northwich. It was two and a half hours from home, and looking after myself was super stressful – my very first household bills. Eek! Still no boyfriend except Andy, sort of, long distance, and I embarked upon an attempt at having the so-called great single life. Supposed to be having the best time of my life, this was the worst time for my loss of control.

▶ *When grub's got a grip on a grown up.*

Don't get me wrong – as any high achiever in a similar situation knows – you can channel your energies as well as the next person so that everyone thinks you're successful and happy. And you probably are – to a certain extent. But when you're a Food Prisoner and grub's got a grip, logic goes out the window. Especially at the end of the day behind closed doors, when the only person you've got to impress is yourself, and you've never understood that bit of life at all.

What is it that makes a self-respecting adult become so controlled by the need to eat that they crave food they can't have, don't stock it so they can't binge on it, but then cave in and leave the house late at night to drive round and round in search of a Topic or a chippy? What is it that makes them choose a best friend who's skinny, albeit as neurotic as I was but for different reasons?

The difference in size between me and my mate, Jax, didn't exactly help me solve the boyfriend dilemma when we went clubbing together. Or on a Scottish skiing holiday where the really attractive ski instructor asked her to dance at the final night 'do' and not me. Not me, the thirteen stone fuchsia pink ski-suited Mrs Blobby hurtling down the ski slopes in a permanent snowplough. Can't understand why he chose her not me … lol. I didn't *really* go back and stuff my face silly that night, *did* I? Not! Lying in bed listening to *99 Red Balloons*, or Go West, or Alison Moyet's *That Ole Devil Called Love*, with my packets of Scottish shortbread and plenty of bags of crisps, I knew I'd hit rock bottom.

I'd hit an all-time high of over thirteen stone by the time I came back and had started to feel the rolls of fat on my back, not just round my waist, but up around my shoulders, too; what a weird thing that was. In later years, I would hit it again, although the next time would be when I was carrying a ten pound baby. At the time, however, I was finally despondent.

11. Emotional Eating

The reasons I eventually ballooned.

The dinner party with the infamous bin-scavenging episode, which I mentioned earlier, happened that spring, I think. Friends from Screensport came to my house and were treated to Spag Bol à la Debbie. They came, they ate, they left some, they went home again. I cleared up, confidently binning the leftovers and leaving the washing up till morning. And went to bed.

So why couldn't I just go to sleep? I'd managed to get as far as chucking the goddam food away – wasn't that enough? Why couldn't those next few hours have passed in a state of satiety, both for food (I'd naturally had over-large portions myself anyway) and for company? And why was I drawn like a magnet to those ample leftovers from skinny people's plates, solidifying into a mass of cold stodge languishing in the bin and calling me from dreamland.

- *'You know we're here!'*
- *'You know your number one rule is never to waste food.'*
- *'You think there'll be a famine tomorrow, you think you have to finish everything off – even other people's leftovers, like there's a war on. Just like when you were at home – the family always cleaned their plates. You were "good" children for eating it all then. You were told you had to eat it all.'*
- *'Yeah, so stop kidding yourself, you know you won't waste it. Just give in, just for today, and come and get us out of this bin – now.'*

After all, it would just be this once and then I'd never do it again, right? So down I went, ate some, and felt totally ashamed and sick of myself the next day.

I'd have been a fully-fledged bulimic but I could never bring myself to throw it up again and waste it. I think the only time I stooped lower than that was when I was determined not to go out in search of food. So I ate everything I could get my hands on within the house, including some old defrosted bits of leftover pastry I'd put in the freezer rather than bear to throw it away. Another error; with Freedom Eating, you can 'waste it' and throw it away rather than force your body to eat it if you've had enough. But back then I was like a woman possessed. Microwaved, soggy and pasty … mmm … a white pastry feast fit for a king – well, for a sad cow in need of some serious help, anyway. And why did this happen so frequently – so much that eventually it became part of the fabric of every day of my life? The answer was obvious, it was emotional eating – comfort eating. I lived alone, I wasn't in a relationship, so I simply fed my pangs of loneliness and angst with food – using all the learned behaviours I'd been adopting for so long.

Soon after, my fortunes changed slightly with a brand new job, and it started to feel like the old days at broadcasting school as I threw myself into my dream job – finally – in radio. I was a broadcast assistant at Piccadilly Radio in Manchester. I was in seventh heaven. The first eight months were a dream time. At last I was in broadcasting and my career was headed in the right direction. Whether as one of Timmy Mallett's helpers (where Chris Evans also began), or vetting Steve Penk's early wind-up callers, I loved every minute of it. Hardly thought about my weight. It was far easier to subsist on ready-meals and fruit. I finally landed an overnight show of my own and a future husband from the sales department called Tony. Tall, dark, handsome, no food problem in sight, he and I hit it off over a badminton court and the rest, as they say is 'His' Story. My story was always fleshed out in private as I fought to deal with my eating problems to a greater or lesser degree.

Hunger for companionship satisfied, I gradually worked my way out of the eating disorders borne of loneliness and stress and pressure on myself to achieve, and by the time we moved back down to London for my new wonder job as Phillip Schofield's replacement and the first female in the Broom Cupboard on Children's BBC, I was regaining some semblance of normality. What are you hungry for, really, when you eat? Is it really the food, or is it something else? It was definitely something else once I was pregnant with my first baby and finishing my stint as a children's presenter before the bump got noticeable. Then another worry took over – I was worried about the future as my contract came to an end, and finding occasional solace in the voice over booth, recording that week's promos whilst munching on a scone and butter, my little 'treat' to myself to keep the morning sickness at bay. Pregnancy kind of took on its own rules about food, flooded as I was with advice and 'instruction' from all and sundry about how not to eat for two.

For the next seven years, I kept my weight down to a healthy ten and a half stone – slim for me and give or take a couple of pounds, the odd post-holiday blowout or a Christmas or a pregnancy, I stayed there. Life was good, albeit Tone and I took it in turns to work, more or less: it always seemed he or I would lose a job or be made redundant in turn. We rarely got to sustain the income, never paid off debts, except with new loans. But we were fine, on the whole. And the kids were great. Although this book might not mention it as much, I tend towards being a happy, contented little soul, and we were doing fine as our little family unit established itself as three, then four, and domestic routine was a welcome break from the pressure to achieve, and part of what became my day to day life.

In September 1990, Lauren was now one year old and I'd got back down to about 10st 5lb. Very slim for me. I felt great, looked fine, and felt good as I did a Dr Who weekend on my current fab job on *31 West* on the satellite service called BSB – remember the squarials? So I can't blame the pregnancies. I could lay a few shovelfuls of blame at the door of comfort eating as a result of Rupert Murdoch's takeover of BSB though. We all got made redundant in the November. Tony and I felt like we were back to square one. I don't think what happened as a consequence of that really ever allowed us to recover from it – we were up and down ever after, really, and so was my helter-skelter of weight loss and gain – till Freedom Eating.

There were some definite highlights, however, during my hunt for more work. I auditioned for a new show called *Stars in Their Eyes* as Sheena Easton – they said 'lose some weight'. I did but not enough, and although I sounded like Sheena Easton, I still looked like Eartha Kitt. But it was great fun to take part in – it's sometimes on YouTube under 'Debbie does Sheena does Eartha!' My weight was then a low, low ten stone two pounds, temporarily through diet pills, diuretic tablets and crash diets, but that was the last time I got to that weight, and, as ever, it was short-lived.

Now I'd like to be that weight again, but the reality is my body might not want to be. If after Freedom Eating away most of the excess pounds, my natural weight is a slightly rounded ten and a half stone, then that's what I'll tend towards, however much I fight it. Another reality check for the terminally hungry.

So along the way there were highs and lows, ups and downs, good times and not so good. Dad dying was a bit of a bummer – another story for another time. But basically it was cancer of the liver in 1992, six months and he was gone. Just like that. It's okay now, I can – and I like to – talk about him fondly, but as everyone knows who's going through bereavement, there aren't any easy answers. Look up 'The Good Grief Trust' if you are, they are very helpful. And on my website there are some recommendations for books and other resources too.

Two years later I landed the job at QVC, the newly launched Shopping Channel in Battersea, London. Great for cash flow, bad for life balance, Zen and 'me-time'. Within another two years I was back up to over eleven stone. Ironically having been very very slim after some painful stressful relationship issues, I began to put on a quarter of a stone every six months. A bread maker here, a cappuccino maker there, all in the name of research. By 1998, I'd reached twelve and a half stone, and so as not to break the pattern, by spring of 1999 I was nearer thirteen, maybe even thirteen and a half. I'd stopped getting on the scales by then. I thought it can't be long before I got to my pre-birth heaviest pregnancy weight. The only difference being I wasn't carrying a ten pounds nine ounces baby. All I needed was a fuchsia pink ski suit and history would have come full circle.

Now a lot of other things happened alongside this continual weight problem, culminating in our first near-miss marriage break up in early 1999. But again, that's another story. Suffice it to say my friends and relations helped me pull through and got me and Tony back on the straight and narrow. For a while anyway ...

And that's maybe what became the catalyst for knowing I had to shake free from the noose of food prison. When having a food problem is pulling you down, you can't think or act straight. When Food Prison's your home, natural body functions can be overridden like a shot, at the prospect of a slap-up meal, a bit of short-lived comfort. Especially when you're not getting what you need elsewhere, in terms of affection, attention or excitement in your life. I'm sure you've all got your own versions.

If your hunger is not really for food, you satiate your needs the only way you know how. The old familiar way that's been with you much of your life – through food. That fleeting pleasure is tangible, if only for a few minutes each time. It's physical. It's controlled by you, it's your decision to go and eat the next thing, and the next, and the next. Because every time is the last time, right? As the experts say when so much in your life is out of your control, no wonder you feel the need to be the one putting yourself consciously in the driving seat at mealtimes, and any time in between. The perfect women's addiction.

In a natural state, our bodies would signal that it's time for us to eat by giving us hunger pangs. Then we'd eat a little, enough for the hunger pangs to stop, till the food tasting so unbelievably good definitely subsides, till we feel comfortable but not so we can feel the food in our belly. Definitely not till we can't breathe any more. We'd eat till we're satisfied. Satisfied. Not full. Not bursting. Then we'd go off and do whatever else we needed to do without another thought about the food. Ideally, food wouldn't be that important – till the next mealtime. But when everything that controls that process is completely imbalanced, when you're used to overriding your body's signals and you tell it when to eat, not the other way round, making it eat when it's not ready for food – like the petrol tank that's not empty yet – the overflow has to go somewhere, and it's usually deposited as fat on the body. How the hell can you have food problems and hope never to have weight trouble? That's the million dollar question – and don't believe anyone who says they have it all sussed.

▶ *So by May 1999, I was ready to change.*

They say when the student is ready the teacher will appear. Never more for me than the first year I found Freedom Eating (commencing in the spring of 1999). Some of the best advice I've ever heard all came along at once. Mostly on various audiobooks. See resources at the back for some I'd recommend, which have most impressed me and impacted in some way on my life. Not just the ones about weight loss specifically, but also about changing, being happy, achieving, communicating and more. They're all part of the same advice really, because until you understand more fully why you do what you do, how can you permanently adopt new behaviours? Information won't change your life. It can help you in understanding yourself and how then to take action in order to make the difference ... this time ... permanently, forever, and for always.

But I'll tell you something, it is possible. Get the right combination of factors together and it's dynamite in your hands.

▶ *You know you're the same as me, in many ways.*

Some may be more pronounced, others less marked. A variation on a theme. Or maybe a carbon copy of where I've come from and what I've been through, which is why I've just included so much of my story so you can see how similar you are to me. And therefore why you can trust me enough to give this system your all. So now I can be your soul mate. Join me here and in our online support groups in a better frame of mind – with a greater understanding – having put the wheel in motion to help things change for the better – permanently. We just have to do it!

12. This Whole Identity Thing

*Powerful visualisations – reclaim
your natural birthright to be slim!*

What makes a woman accept being fat as a part of life? Is it because of the way she's treated? Is it because of what she's told by those around her? Is it because she's basically given up, that she has such a lack of self-worth that she puts up with being less than she deserves to be? Or just that she's kidding herself. How many times do we hear from people who've said that the final straw was 'that photo at the barbecue, with butter running down my chin'. Or 'at the wedding where you couldn't see the bride because as maid of honour I blocked the aisle', or was it someone's comments? Those people who've become slim who still act like they're fat. The way they walk, dress, speak, or their confidence, their beliefs about food. They still comment on everyone else's eating habits, and obviously still have a huge hang-up about the whole food thing. They're in Food Prison, and unless they constantly exercise extreme self-deprivation and control, you just know that one day they're destined to be fat again – to once more grow into the body that fits the image they never grew out of in their mind.

There are also a few fat people who have so much confidence and who are not in food prison, and who grew up with a whole different set of rules surrounding food. Sure, they may like to be slimmer if they could tick a box, but quite frankly they feel okay as they are. Just go to the United States and your average slightly tubby person will feel positively slim comparatively speaking. There are just so many more much-larger people there, unless you're in some parts of California, that even fourteen pounds or so overweight isn't considered big. Not that that helps the likes of you and me when all we've got as a comparison is our own self-image – this year's model, last year's, the year before …

Visualisations

I'm going to take you on a journey into your mind. It's not hypnotism, or anything weird. It's just a basic way of installing a set of images which will help your mind get used to the idea that you can be slim. You can change. One of the biggest driving forces in a human being is the need to be consistent to your own identity, what you believe about who you really are. The dialogue you have about yourself. The words you use, the questions you ask yourself. These visualisation techniques can open up a new realm inside your mind, one where the slim you lays in hiding. Kept there by the resistance to change. It's not just a new wardrobe we're talking about here, it's having to give up all those excuses about your life. Like the woman who, every time she gets close to having to get on with her own life, or face up to sorting out a marriage gone wrong, hides behind having yet another baby. She doesn't really want another baby, in truth she just doesn't want to have to go back to being just herself again. And so it is with the permanently fat person. Here's some food for thought. Think of how overweight you are. Are you usually the same number of pounds overweight? If you manage to keep yourself overweight by a few pounds, it's for a reason.

If you're always overspending the same proportion, no matter what your salary, if you're always late by the same amount of minutes each time, if your house/flat/room is always about the same degree of 'messy', then you're perpetuating certain beliefs about yourself which keep you at that level. Otherwise you'd go far higher, wouldn't you? Chances are, most of the time, you'll be overweight by roughly the same amount. When you're not dieting, and you are 'too fat' by about twenty pounds all the time, it implies that you are capable of maintaining your weight at the same level, you just haven't worked out how to do it at the level you prefer, slightly lower on the scales. Mind you, if someone isn't yet ready for the change to a slimmer image, nothing will help them. If you stay adamant that 'it won't work for me', then guess what, it won't.

I'll keep saying it, one of the biggest driving forces in mankind is to stay consistent with your own identity. Studies which have been done on this subject show that, in general, a person will fight harder not to change than to make change happen. The Inner Chimp doesn't like change. We find it almost impossible to shake our old identity free. We want consistency and certainty. We've been down the route of being fat before and we're used to it. We've got all our fat clothes, our fat lifestyles, our excuses for not walking too far, or for not having a man. We know our fat image like a comfort blanket and we're sticking to it. We like our comfort zones. We prefer the status quo.[10]

Making things different is hard to cope with, which is why forming new habits is so much harder than breaking old ones. The first four weeks of the new fitness routine, or giving up smoking, or getting those essays done on time and so much more. They're all much harder than the twenty fourth week, or the eleventh month, or the sixtieth year. So what can we do to help ourselves accept a new identity and act accordingly? Lots of things – visualisations especially, can help enormously, as a part of the overall transformation.

Imagine yourself in twenty years' time. What if you've never changed those habits? What if you've stayed in food prison? What if all your photos, and videotapes from all those holidays in all those years had you looking the way you don't want to look – fat – according to you at least? I'll say 'fat' because there will be some of you who make everyone sick because you look great but you just *think* you're fat. Others would die to look just like you, but nevertheless, you perceive yourselves to have a food problem, to not be able to eat normally. Perhaps the only reason you are decent-looking to other people is because you've taken up permanent residence in food prison and refuse to come out. You've thrown away the key. But little do you realise that you could still keep your shape, even lose a little more maybe, if you gave up this addictive identity – this habit – and put something else in its place. If you formed new associations. New associations with your shape. A few pounds or a little roll around your middle is not 'I'm fat'. If you formed new associations with your eating habits and with other people's eating habits and with food in general, you would be given the key to a much happier life. And there are others like you too. (See the guises of Freedom Eater later.) As for the rest of you who probably, or definitely, *are* fat, well imagine this, let your mind really run riot with this one for at least five minutes and get your feelings down on paper if you can. Literally – get a pen and a piece of paper.

Imagine if you had the key out of this food prison now; this year or even this month. Someone somewhere is going to come and teach you how to be a slim person and how to eat like one, think like one and act like one. Release yourself and those around you from all the hang-ups that food prisoners base their lives around. Would you pay big bucks for it? You bet you would! It would be on the bestseller list immediately.

Isn't that why so many so-called wonder cures, miracle-diets, latest food fads, diet trends, pills, potions, lotions, machines, operations, books, clubs, courses and diet foods are always so popular? But they never work permanently. What kind of industry is this that deals solely with the symptoms of a problem, and never truly get to grips with what's stopping it from providing a permanent solution? A profitable one! How many new diet books were released and sold last year, the year before and the decade before that? If you kept taking your car to a garage for the same repair over and over again in the course of your life, and every time you questioned what they were doing they blamed your driving, you'd begin to wonder if the garage really knew what it was doing, wouldn't you? You bet you would. Well, it's the same with the diet industry. So you need never blame yourself again – ever – for not sticking to that rigid diet you swore blind was going to be the last ever one, because they don't work permanently. Dieting is now believed to actually lower your metabolic rate so much that your body then needs even fewer calories than it did before in order to reach the point at which it starts storing them up as fat.

▶ *So dieting can actually make you fatter.*

Your body was born with a genetically predetermined bone structure, ideal weight and height distribution. Your predetermined weight is called your *set point*. Your body goes to great lengths to defend this designed weight, which is your *ideal body weight* – not *your* ideal, but your *body's* ideal, whether *you* like it or not. Your body makes it very difficult to lose below this weight and for some, very difficult to gain above this weight. It does this by raising or lowering your basal metabolic rate, which is the rate your body burns calories while at rest. Dieting can reduce the metabolic rate by 15–40%, whereas forced feeding can increase the rate in some people by as much as 75%.[11] In one study, volunteers were fed double their usual intake over a six-month period, with the goal of increasing their weight by 20% – 25%. Although the first few pounds were gained easily, the total weight gained was 75% less than expected, based on intake, due to the fact that their metabolic rate increased.[12]

▶ *We all know what to do. We just don't do what we know. It's the 'why' that this book is all about.*

So how can the visualisation help? Why don't you start with some nice 'me-time'? I want you to find some soft music – background music, not strong melodies – and give yourself five minutes of 'me-time'. Get a pen and notebook, a journal style one if possible, so you can keep all your thoughts together. As Tony Robbins says, 'If your life's worth living, it's worth recording.'[13] I agree, just don't get all anal about it. There's nothing worse than the feeling that you 'have to' do something. If you don't want to, don't do it! On the other hand, if you find you want to write for four hours and fill it front to back, then feel free to do that too: Freedom Living, remember? The great thing is, this process is just for you. No one else will need to see it or read it unless you want them to. You may want to show someone special in order to help you make it more real – it's your call.

Now with the music playing, just write. Don't think about it too much, or stop, or think what you should be writing, just write, and get to the bottom of what it's really like to be fat. Your life, now. How does being fat hold you back, embarrass you and stop you from fulfilling your potential? Feel it, live it, write it. Visualise and record all this then you can *change it*. Write as much as you feel is inside you. Have some tissues ready just in case it all gets a bit emotional. For some people it will, for some it won't, there's no right or wrong, okay?

When you've done that, for now, think yourself forward whilst you're in this mode. What's life going to be like in five years' time if you don't make the changes? How will it affect your life, and the people around you? What will you miss out on? Now it gets even more intense. Think yourself forward ten years to what your life will be like if you haven't made the changes. Keep the music going, the same music for all of this thinking forward bit. You'll need a different more uplifting music in a minute. I think you can guess what's coming. When you're right in the middle of visualising you in twenty years' time – the worst of it, if you never made the changes, I want you to make the first change and as soon as you're finished and ready for the next stage, change the music over.

Now remember, everything you just wrote hasn't happened yet – it can be different, it's not too late. It's just like someone's given you another chance to re-do the next twenty years. None of what you described has to come to pass – yet. You've got the opportunity to make a difference, if it starts right now. So now describe what you would be like – in the present initially, if you did start to make the changes you know are needed. Don't leave out any details. What would you feel like? How would people react differently to you? How confident would you be? Put it all down.

Now do the same again – for five and then ten years' time and think – how different would your life be if you broke out of Food Prison? Fill yourself with that joyous feeling that you'd get if you knew it was all going to happen, and now do one last thing. Notice all the conditionals in what you've just written – should, would, could, if. Now I want you to re-write it as if it was true right now. As if your fairy godmother had wafted in with her wand and her hobnail boots and instantly given you your desires. 'I am slim and beautiful. I am fit and active. I use the stairs instead of the lift. I walk the dog every morning before work. I never overeat. I always listen to my body. I am a size twelve skirt.' If you want, these can be affirmations, or incantations, or your own code of conduct, whatever you want to call it. There are many different perceptions of this process. Louise Hay and Bernie Siegel talk about affirmations in their work.[14] Good old Tony Robbins calls the future you technique, The Dickens Process (ghosts of Christmas future, present and past), and goes into this method more fully at his excellent Unleash the Power Within/Life Revolution weekends around the world, including Wembley in London, Frankfurt in Germany and in the US, where you also get the chance to do a firewalk – I've done two and they are wonderful metaphors for overcoming the barriers in your beliefs. Otherwise his books and audiobooks give lots more detail as to how these and other techniques can help you in your transformation.[15] Use it if it works for you too. Other experts have their own versions too – there's tons out there. Go google.

And if you're a real old-school sceptic, a cynic of the first degree, then do whatever part of this feels comfortable to you. Opening up your mind to some of this latest psychology can in itself be a giant leap and not one you can make readily or instantly, so again, don't worry about it. I only ask you to test the theory not necessarily to instantly believe. And if you can change the way you feel about your image, your identity, your self-belief and references, even a chink, then you may have to just re-think about who you are and what you stand for. Even if it's only a tiny change you make every time you sit down to think about it, then all those little changes will soon add up to be a big change, and you'll definitely be taking yourself onto a different path.

Do you know the best thing about Freedom Eating? It's just this – it's allowing you to reclaim your natural birthright to be slim. Now go back into your past. If you can remember a time when you had no thought of food and were a normal weight, and you didn't worry about food the whole time, even if you occasionally considered cutting down a bit, or were conscious that you shouldn't eat too much chocolate in one go, back when you are one of the lucky ones. Anyone can go back to the state you were born in, being able to naturally control what food your body needed to eat. You just have to do one thing. One thing. It's a big one.

▶   *Trust your body.*

It doesn't come naturally, but it's something, which once you've started doing, will be as easy as breathing. Because it makes sense. Because it's not contrived. Because it's not depriving yourself. Because it's not going to make you get bored with it. Because it's not hard. Because it makes food even more enjoyable than it ever was before in your life. Because you see results. Because it's liberating. Because let's face it, it's easy. Babies can do it and toddlers can do it, if they haven't already been indoctrinated by contrived socialisation. Deprivation and control can kick in from a very early age, just look at some of the obese pre-school kids. Especially the ones whose mothers are huge or who fill them up with sugar, fruit juice or processed rubbish. Or even 'healthy' bars full of fructose.

It's all gone wrong mainly in the last few hundred years, but more particularly, for those of us alive now, since the Second World War. Rationing is to blame. Rationing mentality has never really gone away. No wonder, if it's an intrinsic and powerful part of our grandparents' child-rearing and has therefore been handed down and become part of everyday life for us. And if it's good enough for us, it's got to be good enough for our children. Why does it perpetuate itself so much? Because we don't learn how to be parents from anyone else but those who bring us up. So what they do, by and large, we do. Oh sure, the brand of nappy, and the toys and pastimes may evolve, but why would it ever occur to you to change the habits we teach regarding food and mealtimes, when we don't even realise they're wrong? For decades now we've been propounding the same myths to do with food and eating. Telling ourselves, and our children, the same stories. Even as I sat in a hotel in Spain with my laptop, writing this chapter originally, the words I heard at lunchtime were resounding in my ears. My son left two potato croquettes on his plate. He'd finished. For me, that's a reason to rejoice! My mum's then partner, Tom, however, didn't have a clue.

- *'Why don't you eat those other two, Brad? No point leaving them.'*
- *'I've finished.'*
- *'But there's only two, they're only small, eat them, they're lovely.'*
- *'No.'*

End of conversation. Thank goodness. My son is now in the world of the slim people. And though he may at times stuff himself with Maltesers and eat four packets of crisps, he is in touch with his body as much as the next slim person.

Again at the time of writing this chapter originally, my daughter told me, since we were having this conversation, that Daddy still used to ask her to finish what was on her plate. When they were out having a meal not long beforehand, she told him, 'I don't feel like it,' and he replied, 'Oh rubbish!' Ever heard that one before? Ever done that one before? How on earth anyone can second guess what another person feels is beyond me! He should definitely know better by now. But he'll get used to it. As Wayne Dyer says to the people who try to insist he acts as they want him to act. 'You want me to do it your way? You think I'm wrong? You'll get over it.'[16]

The best thing we can do for our children is never comment on body shapes or criticise their eating in relation to a part of their anatomy. The days of, 'What are you eating that for, you'll get fat as an old pig,' have long ceased to be a problem for me. It still amuses me somewhat that my mother will still say, 'What are you eating now?' But if I just remind myself that it usually happens when she's back at slimming club and is feeling the deprivation and control more markedly than usual in her own life, it helps me recognise the place she's in, and just let it go. The need for retribution is useless in the quest to understand your own body and its foibles, and smiling sweetly and just acknowledging the critic's comments but ignoring them and not letting it affect you, can often get the message across more effectively than ever trying to waste time explaining it all, or worse – arguing. Vikki told me at the start of all this that other people will learn when they are ready, and there's no point trying to get them into the Freedom Eating ethic until they want to know. Never a truer word. I have had great success with my sister, who now understands the principles behind it a little more, but is presently some way off from true Freedom Eating, because she prefers to combine it with dieting, and that's okay too. (See the 'When' Diet later.)

The critics will get there – when they're ready and they will join the thousands around the world finally breaking free from Food Prison into a brave new world. Ironically, the same world we would have lived in our entire lives had social conditioning and learned behaviour, habits and deprivation and control not interfered.

So once you've mastered the art of changing your own image of yourself and not living up to the expectations of those around you who may put you off, you will be ready to help those people when they see the change in you and want some of it for themselves. They'll be ready for Freedom Eating.

13. A Very Difficult Period

When life gets in the way.

The original *Till the Fat Lady Slims* in 2002 was about following Full Freedom Eating, i.e., following the 'When' Diet (see later) Principles One to Six, but giving yourself full freedom of choice and no restrictions – otherwise combine it with a traditional diet. I do full Freedom Eating and cannot diet for the life of me. But one element works for both.

The question, 'Do I really want it?' is a really powerful one, especially for someone who's been living their life according to ingrained habits for years and years. That was me, when I began writing the original book.

I was married when I started writing it, and it transversed one of the most traumatic periods in my life as I ended up getting divorced in between finishing the original book and it going to press. There then followed a period of transition – major transition – so pull up a chair. Gulp. Off we go.

We all have a story – and this chapter covers the era of my life where I coped with:

- Becoming a single mum.

- Getting used to being divorced.

- Starting up a whole business empire and seeing it crumble again.

- Being made redundant four times in two years – serves me right for working in the finance industry. An ex-boyfriend ran a – yes you've guessed it – sub-prime mortgage company. Eeek! I'm coming out in hives just thinking about it …

- … and about him. It wasn't a good period in my life, and I went through treatment for depression. And out the other side again.

- Through it all, in those early years, my kids were relying on me – solely me – to get them through their teenage years and university. Which I did. Alone. How brilliant.

- I had a couple of other boyfriends – including a 'tragically funny one night stand'. It was so funny, in fact, that it made it into one of my romance novels, as a never-to-be-repeated experience for the heroine, Sadie. Another relationship I had in the early 2010s started out with the guy declaring loudly he was a single man, yet he still pursued me, so 'Debbie the rescuer' clicked into 'fix him' mode – he was someone with issues, with cheese and cats. And money. And authority. And staying positive and hopeful. Unfixable. *Eurgh.*

- Plus a house move which precipitated an excruciatingly awful declutter, stressful beyond belief, along with the realisation that I was moving into a house that was just for me alone ... *a house which turned out to be a nightmare for three glaring reasons.*

Needless to say, I have totally learned from these experiences and view myself now as a wiser individual. And still ever hopeful of finding the right man to settle down with. 'One day ...' you know the rest, '*When I'm a grown up!*'

Just when you're not looking ...

Oh yes, I had my fair share of 'What was I thinking' eras. And it took its toll on my well-being. In this chapter I've decided to go into more detail about the whys and wherefores of what happened to me after I first wrote about Freedom Eating up until I began a whole new focus on fitness and health with a new website blog. Much of the 2000s and some of the 2010s.

Later, you'll even find a short outline of my own ideal routine to get in shape – for those who really want to be guided – I've called it the 'Debbie-F (that's me) Plan' diet! Hehe! Read on ...

What happened 2000–2002

It was a funny time in my life, this one. I remember talking to a friend, Ali, about what she called my 'metamorphosis'. All the while I was writing the original *Till the Fat Lady Slims*, I was actually going through a painful marriage break-up.

I ended up finding out that after fourteen years, The Man and I had different ideas of what it took to make a marriage work. A year after we split up, I discovered he'd been playing around – for most of our marriage, as it happens. Seriously. Whilst I had been completely faithful.

The one thing it did do was to give me the peace of mind that through it all, when I used to have suspicions, they were actually correct. So I knew I could trust my instincts after all.

At that time, I was learning a lot about myself. I thoroughly recommend a lot of resources if you need to do the same – self-help books and audio books – from Wayne Dyer to Tony Robbins, Deepak Chopra to business books like Steven Covey and Kenneth Blanchard. *The 7 Habits of Highly Effective People* was one of my favourites, as 'seek first to understand then be understood' became one of my mantras. There's a whole list on my website.[17]

As did Wayne Dyer's 'give up your need to be right,' and 'be independent of the good and bad opinion of others'. His way of dealing with people who disagree vehemently with your choices, changed my life at that point. For instance, when someone close to me told me they didn't approve of a purchase I'd just made, or what I was doing with my life, I'd just reply, 'You'll get over it.' Dealing with those moments more efficiently makes such a difference to your peace of mind – making me more able to carry on with my job of changing the habits of a lifetime. It's a hard one to master though, 'cos the 'tribe' don't like it when a member steps outside the box.

Don't be scared to counter their objections. When you start saying 'Actually I don't feel like it,' or 'Not now, but I'd love to save one for later,' it will irk some people. But they'll get used to it …

Some people around me were initially sarcastic and took the mick. Especially people who poo-poo most things – you know, the bitter ones, or the life-long cynics. Or the ones who purport to know it all, but never practise what they preach. But this time there was one big difference – they soon changed their tune when they saw how my body was slimming down more easily than ever before. Finally, here was a 'diet' that worked. Only Freedom Eating is not a diet. It's about as opposite from a controlled diet as you can get. I loved this time in my life for that reason, even if my marriage was falling apart.

I realised there was no point trying to change their minds, not if they clearly were not ready to listen. But proving by actions not words that things really were different eventually made those very people curious. They would sidle up and casually ask how I'd done it, especially when I lost weight over Christmas one year. That was a big 'Aha' moment in my life – it is in most people's lives actually.

I'd had enough … my last married Christmas

I guess I finally discovered I needed to live my life without obeying his rules, after all. And of course Ex-Husband-To-Be didn't accept that very easily. Previously I'd cave in to a situation, so that he'd get his way and I'd just go smother my emotion with food. Gradually it became the norm that I no longer caved in. Gradually I began to not accept things for an easy life, and I began to properly challenge his demands, standing up for myself instead. I decided to battle to fix what was at the heart of the problem – the problem that previously caused my married emotional eating.

Initially my independence was admired by him, and he was seemingly proud of what I was doing to change my shape – after all, he'd always kept himself trim and fit so it was something he admired. But insidiously over the years he seemed to become snooty about my opinions. But then came Freedom Eating. The differences of opinion about the kids and their mealtimes really came under scrutiny. I began getting everyone to sit down at the table with me, rather than in front of the telly. I'd say 'okay' if they told me they'd had enough, whereas his reaction was a throwback to his (and my) childhood – 'Finish what's on your plate.' 'No,' I'd say, 'if they've had enough it's okay to leave it.' And at the same time, he'd started staying out at 'work' longer and longer, until our marriage reached breaking point once I moved up to Peterborough half the week for a new job.

Yes, I left QVC. BUT in this brave new world of being completely independent again, I was ruling my own life, with no one else to worry about for half the week – the other half I was back down in the family home again, as that was the deal after we'd split up.

I'd go to Frankie and Benny's diner on the estate near where the new job was based for lunch with some of the team, and obey the Slim Person's credo, epitomised by Freedom Eating. Consequently I'd end up obeying my deep breath and stopping at satisfied, bringing home half the chicken, salad and chips to eat later. Leftovers became 'de rigueur!' People soon got used to me.

I got used to me.

And I liked me.

I carried on losing the weight, and ended up being more slim and toned, pushing forty, than I had been for most of my thirties. In fact, at thirty-six I'd been my heaviest ever, and desperately unhappy. I knew at that time that I was an emotional eater – the 'binge' I describe later in this book really happened. Some of you may not believe it – looking back now, I hardly believe it myself! How much food I ate at one sitting was scary. But it was indeed happening – frequently, and all behind closed doors. So having left that person behind, I was damned if I was going to slip back again without a fight. A fight that took on a new lease of life when I attended one particular seminar.

Whilst up in Peterborough in the early 2000s I went on a life-changing series of workshops by Tony Robbins.[18] His stuff is still pretty mind-blowing, if you like that sort of thing. Yes, it's all a bit happy-clappy, but I was embracing it all back then – in truth it was exactly what I needed.

I went to his others – Hawaii, on 'Life Mastery' and to Miami on 'Date with Destiny' and both these week-long workshops helped me grasp a much better understanding of how I tick. If you are interested in future workshops then just look him up.

So another thing I can take out of that era is that, if you want to change the habits of a lifetime, it won't be overnight. But with the right techniques, new habits can be formed. And a supportive environment is vital to enable you to continue the journey and not slip back to old ways.

In fact, it took me another few years, until a major upset in my life, for any slipping to occur.

Bad business – 2002–2009

After a couple of years of being single, I'd pretty much got a grip on my new life. At the end of the day, when the doors closed and the lights went off, I was as guilty as the next person of sitting listening to sad songs and hosting my own private pity party, à la Bridget Jones. But at least I'd stopped bingeing – in fact, I've never binged again since discovering Freedom Eating, as I explain in the Binge Management section later on.

But that's not to say a marriage break-up didn't hit me hard, 'cos it did. I remember when *Bridget Jones's Diary*, the movie, came out. I saw it with a friend who declared, 'That's you!' over and over again through the film. I had to laugh at the bit where poor thirty-something singleton Bridget feels sorry for herself, singing *All by Myself*. My Whitney Houston CD got a pretty good bashing that year, I can tell you. But happily, shortly after that I was off to Hawaii. It was there that my life changed and I encountered a whole new business opportunity, which kicked off a brand new era in my life and a brand new me. I discovered Penta Water.

Now if you read *Take a Chance on Me*, my first romance novel, you'll know that Sadie the heroine ends up running a special bottled water business. Well, it's not all fiction – the water bit, anyway. Sadie getting off with the millionaire investor was definitely all made up – sadly! But much of the basis of how the water helped performance was inspired by the Penta Water story. I first encountered it on sale on a little table outside the main conference hall at the Hilton Waikoloa, during Life Mastery in Hawaii.

Two years later, in 2002, I had an embryonic importing business, but was still dabbling in shopping telly at another channel – I'd left Peterborough now. In an ideal world I'd have stayed. But I discovered it wasn't one.

The big leap to running my own business full-time came with a canny connection from our short-term PR guru whom we'd met when I was at the previous shopping channel. We'd hired him to help get us some publicity – which included Chris Evans and TGI Friday actually mentioning what we were all getting up to – laughing at our attempts to stay on air by selling autographed photos of ourselves – well, we didn't have enough products but we had the crew and the manpower to stay on air, as long as we were 'selling' something! In former years that kind of stress would have ended up with me drowning my anxiety in the biscuit tin, for sure, but thanks to Freedom Eating, I worked my way through it all, including a very stressful parting of the ways with said channel.

Anyway, the PR guru put me in touch with another of his clients, who had used his PR firm successfully for his big sports company and it turned out he was a venture capital investor. This guy was really interested in Penta after he found out it helped him avoid jet lag, and with his financing and encouragement, along with a wise financial advisor he put in place called Philip, the fledgling Penta UK was up and running. I was in and out of inconsequential relationships at that time, having quite a good time on online dating, to be frank! But I was really slim, for me, and at least I had my crucial master plan – next year we'd all be millionaires! Not really, but at least with a sound business plan and some proper bank financing and all the usual things that go with retailing, I had a genuine prospect of making some serious money if we could tie down the exclusive contract for the UK.

Hopes, dream, plans – you know the stuff. I had them all. I was working in and out of other shopping channels for a couple of years too, 'jobbing around the industry' as they say, but Penta UK represented my future. Or so I thought.

By early 2004 we had offices in Leatherhead, a small team of six or so, two business partners, about five hundred retail outlets in the UK (Waitrose came later), and enough finance for me to go full-time. Our investor wanted proper marketing advice, so we employed a fabulous marketing company, who in turn put me in touch with a guy called Harry, CEO of a successful energy drinks brand. Harry became my mentor and I loved every second of being in charge of this embryonic potential gold mine. I was too busy to be lonely and the last thing on my mind was to resort to emotional eating. By now it almost became anathema to do so.

Mark, my sports director, was expertly bringing on sports teams and athletes, boat race crews and premier football teams, as well as top rugby clubs and celebrities, who all *paid for* our special performance water, by the way. Even Tom Cruise was pictured with a Penta in his hand. The science behind it was impressive, and by early 2005 we'd achieved an amazing feat – three UK universities did early studies which showed our water was definitely different and agreed to go on to full-scale research for us. We were poised for something magnificent.

Through it all, I'd maintained my Freedom Eating – and stayed roughly the same weight.

Yes, there were stressful times, but healthy eating was absolutely my body's default choice. In fact, after a short period of three months being vegan in 2000 for one of the Tony Robbins workshop challenges, I'd noticed how much better my body felt. For several years after that I did mainly 'clean' eating – mostly veggie, and very few unhealthy foods, sweets, etc., as the signals from my body were that I just didn't want them. Plus, of course, lots of water! I was almost never ill. More importantly, our sales went from strength to strength and I was the sweetheart of the manufacturing company based in San Diego, holding business meetings, PR meetings, overseeing contracts, hiring staff and obviously still being a single mother. The dream of what was to be kept me going. After all, we're never so happy as when we are dreaming about future happiness, right?

Then things started to fall apart

We were under big pressures to perform, under our new exclusive contract, which we'd managed to obtain. Harry had helped impress the US parent company that manufactured Penta, and him coming with me along with our investor to meet them all in San Diego had sealed the deal – we were now the UK and Europe distributor. We had begun making some dramatic inroads in UK press and newspapers and amongst sportsmen and women. Penta was really working.

BUT – do you recall the Dasani bottled water debacle, around 2004? Bottled purified city water? It made people wary of expensive water that needed an explanation, whereas previously it hadn't even been an issue. The scientific patented process was hard to explain, and the UK university full studies were not yet concluded. Our sales faltered. Then the parent company decided to tighten up their contract terms, as our sales weren't high enough. And without going into too much detail, as that's a book in itself, we floundered. I had one of the most painful periods of my whole life and not only at work – at home, the kids had reached exam stage too and finances were tougher and tougher.

By mid 2005, we had no alternative but to wind up the business. And with it, all the personal investment I'd made, meaning I too went bankrupt. There wasn't much option for an alternative and believe me I looked for another way. But with the blessing of our investor, we dissolved the company. He was a rock, and still is – we meet for coffee every so often even now. And, yes, he's read my novel, *Take a Chance on Me*, and no, he doesn't seem bothered that the hero is based on him. And Daniel Craig.

But things looked bleak for me, financially. It was one of the most stressful times of my life, that's for sure.

At the same time, my boy was doing his A-levels, and getting ready to go to uni, and my girl was doing her GCSEs and moving to college. So whilst I was putting a brave face on it on the outside, I was hurting inside, big time, and my focus got a little off target.

There was a little light at the end of the tunnel, or so I thought, in the form of a 'rescuer' relationship. A new guy. A boyfriend – one who was the MD of a mortgage company, who worked in the same serviced offices as we did. We met to discuss our companies, swap advice, etc., and he was funny, witty, clearly intelligent and driven. It was clear he liked me. Later he admitted bringing in his bike just so I could see him in his cycling gear, and sneaking into the offices after hours to sniff my cardigan which I left on the back of my chair. Weird. He said it with a smile so I just laughed and decided to consider it flattering. Rather than weird. Shame I hadn't learned to trust my gut back then. The importance of gut was to come a decade later.

When he split from his wife of one year, he came straight to me, that night, and I gladly accepted him, having previously refused to be party to any form of cheating. After all, I'd been on the receiving end of infidelity myself courtesy of Ex-Husband so I didn't want to inflict it on another woman. The clue to its fate might have been in the 'that night' part though …

Mr Mortgage and I forged ahead with a relationship, but I knew so early on it was doomed. To be honest, admitting it for the first time here, he made being with him very difficult but little by little my self-regard was eroded. He even kicked out at me in bed one night when I got in next to him at his flat and put my cold feet on his leg. What an idiot I was for not just walking away right there. He also had several tantrums when we were out with family and friends, once even sending me – and my fifteen-year-old daughter Lauren – to 'Coventry' when we had a day out at Hampton Court, and frequently letting me down when he was supposed to be joining in with family activities. He was one of those men who was okay in a crowd, holding court, as I used to call it. I used to quite like it when he did that actually. But not with my family – an only child, he had no frame of reference for family, hated Christmas and was more bothered about money and his company than anything else. BUT I was blind to the damaging effect I was letting it have on my own sanity.

I just didn't have the resources to cope with giving him up alongside everything else going wrong. He threw money at my problems, which frankly was a short-term solution and a long-term disaster. It didn't help my state of mind. I'd always been independent and it emasculated me. Which sounds strange, but considering I'd been the mum AND the dad for several years, and fiercely independent, it was making me feel useless to rely on someone else in that way. But I took that road as an easy option, partly to avoid another argument with him, which only made me feel worse. I didn't have much choice, not with Lauren still at home, watching her hapless mother conduct a love affair with a man eleven years my junior and who was blatantly obviously not right for me. She laughs about it now, but I was far from laughing at the time. I was bitterly, bitterly unhappy but unable to cope and coupled with my business going down the pan, and bankruptcy, I didn't realise it but I was sinking into a depression.

Mr Mortgage and I split up five times in the first year. And in just under two years, we had ever-more violent break ups, some ending in bruises on my face – there, I've said it. We split up twelve times in all. It's too long a story for this book, and it's not entirely relevant to the theme. But I'm just setting the scene so you can understand how this major upheaval in my life led to my next phase. At one point he even told me I looked old and ugly – I'd started to give in to his demands for not obeying my body at mealtimes and amidst the feeling down, it seemed a small price to pay for peace. He and I parted twenty-two months after we began, and about eighteen months later than we should have done.

By then I'd been working for him, and that job ended too.

My world kind of fell apart – all my own fault but it was made worse by being a victim of circumstance somewhat. And the word 'victim' and 'me' had never been in the same sentence. But fate dealt its hand, and if everything happens for a reason, I was damn sure I didn't know what it was at that time. I'd learned some major lessons, but was left being treated for depression.

14. Dealing with Depression – 2006

Yes, depression. Me.

No, I wouldn't have believed it either. But there it was, a little blister pack of Citalopram, small dose, taking me through six months I'd rather not ever repeat again in my life. They served a purpose, those little pills. Gave me some wicked adventure type dreams! There was no low, but there was no high either. It eventually took about another two years to fully get them out of my system. They definitely mucked up my brain chemistry. And put me in what I called 'citalopram neutral', where nothing made me desperately sad any more, but nothing made me wonderfully happy either. Weird time.

When I'd begun my relationship with Mr Mortgage, amidst his talk of marriage and not wanting to have babies 'cos I already had them – what a load of tosh as he was married with two children a few years later – I found myself being bullied again, in the same way Ex-Husband had done years before. Only this time round I'd kind of lost sight of myself. With diminished confidence, I didn't have enough fight in me, and I began to get out of the habits of my precious Freedom Eating.

Mr Mortgage would moan if I wasn't ready to eat when he'd made me dinner. He'd also want desserts and expect me to join in. He'd frequently make food his 'thing' and what with the tragic nature of our on/off relationship, my patterns of eating began to change. There's more to it than that – far more – but you get the idea.

After we ended, and my business had folded completely, I went off to work for another mortgage company, then another. Yes, they were sub-prime mortgage packagers. My new career was back in finance, where I'd begun, having taken a business degree at the London School of Economics to become a chartered accountant. So it wasn't a massive mismatch. Ironically I thoroughly enjoyed it.

At the time it was my lifeline – safe. A routine-based daily grind, which gave me regular as clockwork hours and roles – was just what I needed in the midst of my depressed years, back then. Heck, I even found the highlight of my day was making my cup of tea with sugar in (lots) which I frequently made myself and drank throughout my working day. I managed a team of more than a dozen mortgage processors and found myself learning the ins and outs of obtaining mortgages for people with less than perfect credit profiles. People like me.

I wasn't myself at all during that period.

I recall one weekend when the kids were busy and I was at a loss for what to do with myself. I ended up deciding that the thing that would give me more pleasure than anything else was to go back into work, armed with my manager's set of keys, and newly purchased bleach and cloths, and spend my Saturday afternoon an hour away in our Caterham offices, completely cleaning out the grimy communal kitchen. Yes, really. That was probably quite a low point in my life, I must say. The kitchen looked nice though!

Coupled with that, I was slowly getting used to the typical office way of life. My lovely ladies would bring in home-made cakes. The wonderful mortgage lenders whom we worked with would send in tins of sweets every time a big deal came off. And it was always someone's birthday or event.

Gradually the weight crept back on.

I didn't notice it at first, but it hit home one time when I had a tragically funny one-night stand. I was quite large again by the time this happened. I had come through four redundancies in three years, from various sub-prime mortgage companies as they folded one-by-one. I was just back working in media. That had happened via deciding to retrain for a different career, by obtaining Prince 2 professional operations management qualifications, which is used for Operations Managers in, for example, big charities, construction industry, the health service and others, but what it led to was a job as a manager at another shopping channel! They had me back on air by Christmas. It was like shopping telly saying, 'You can't escape meeeee!'

During my year working for Sit-Up – yes I know, same as in Bridget Jones! – I decided to try to give dating another go. I was back amongst 'my people' and feeling very much more myself. It wasn't the best environment – not many places are, it seems. My male manager counterparts were so unable to deal with their female employees – usually the assistant presenters – bursting into tears on a regular basis, that they kept 'score' marks on the whiteboard like notches on the wall, showing how often each of them had made someone cry. They didn't all do it, but it made me roll my eyes! Disciplinary offences nowadays, I'm sure.

Anyway, I was working my way through this baptism of fire when I stumbled across an old flame on the internet. I'd remembered this guy from my days as a drama student and he was loooovely back then. All tall with great cheekbones and brown eyes and floppy brown hair. Well, it turned out he was now like an Iggy Pop version of his former self, performing in a group and we got back in touch via his website. We met up, he was apparently with someone, but it was ending, he said. I went to say goodbye after quite a nice chat and a bit of reminiscing, but he ended up snogging me at the end of the night, and some of the old magic was there. One night he came back to mine for dinner and we ended up in bed again – like old times. With one awful difference. I had a problem with my pelvic floor, after big, big children and weight loss ups and downs. Yes, you can imagine. And he was quite fit, cycling everywhere, and we had a very 'energetic' bedroom session. However, due to his use of weed, I found out later, it wasn't a very 'fulfilling' one. I can describe this in more detail but instead I need you to use your imagination – lots of different positions none of which really worked for his faltering manhood and all the while me trying not to pee myself. Yes, really.

Experiences are never wasted though and it led to a particularly tragic love scene for one of my heroines in one of my novels. Although I held back on some of the detail. That's definitely for another book!

But I was very down on myself afterwards, feeling embarrassed about my body. So shortly afterwards I had surgery.

I had time off for a mini op on my waterworks, two weeks of sitting still, reading, eating and recovering. It was followed soon after by my first writing workshop – in Tuscany, eating amazing food but too much pasta and desserts, and late night snacks as we all learned about 'show not tell' and sub-plots and head hopping. I came back pretty big. Again. I'd never resumed binge eating, that was one blessing. And on the flip side, I'd finally managed to work my way back to QVC.

Every year since I left, someone from QVC had called me to ask if I could go back. And every year, I'd say, 'Yes, of course, speak to you next year,' – as nothing ever happened, since the old MD was dead set against it since several of us had left in such a public way and set up a competitor back in 2000. Can't blame him, really. This particular year, however, he had retired and they definitely needed people who could hit the ground running. So I got 'the call'. 'Can you come back and be a guest, we've got permission and you can definitely come back this time,' they said. But I was on air at another channel at that point, so this was the only year – the first and only year – that I had to say, 'No, I can't be a guest as I'd get the sack. But if you want me back as a presenter then the answer is yes!'

No surprise then, that finally, after nine years away, I managed to visualise hard enough that the powers that be at QVC decided it was time for me to return.

15. Back at QVC, Back to Me, 2009–2014

I was home.

After all my years away, having seen my two kids off to uni and having had major ups and downs, I was back in the fold. But things had changed. Whilst over half of the people were ones I knew, the other half hadn't even heard of me, and the systems were different and, worst of all, my reputation preceded me.

I'd always been ambitious and when I came back, I was told by the then-boss (who left shortly after) that I had to accept a lower wage but 'if I proved myself' and upped sales, I could expect a big increase within a couple of years. So I went hell for leather using all the things I had learned when away from QVC at more difficult channels, all the things that I could see were missing from my time there previously. And no surprise, became a bit unpopular with some of the crew! That didn't help my ability to chuck down the calories and fat grams and all those other methods of counting, which were anathema to the Freedom Eating me!

In the next five years, I was to learn the amazing science about how bad sugar is – which we all take for granted now, don't we! (See later.) I was also to uncover different guises of Freedom Eater as the new social media platforms allowed me to set up a supremely successful support system online. (More about that later as well.) But for now, I was suckered into old habits. I knew I had to do something, but what? By now I was back at QVC four days a week, full pelt. It was lovely doing Thornton's chocolate hours, or eating delicious yogurts for a whole hour, but I'd got too far removed from the basic principles of Freedom Eating. And there lay the problem. I realised it was probably sugar. I had got pretty unfit too. So I had to do something that worked …

A weight loss programme called Diet Chef helped and I lost a stone, and if you do what it says, it works. But for me, as you've probably guessed, I have trouble with the 'doing what it says' bit. So I put it gradually back on again. Sure, those systems work – they work for many who can follow a plan – and if you can too, that's great. Or, if you quite like following a plan but need extra help, or you'd like it to feel easier, well that's where the 'When' Diet comes in – just do both concurrently. (I explain how later on.)

But I still personally can't diet. As I keep saying, if someone tells me 'you can't', it's like a red rag to a bull – because then I want to – whatever 'it' is, even if I didn't want to beforehand.

By summer 2011 my daughter had finished uni and announced she was staying in Bath and wouldn't be moving back home any more. I'd got into the habit of feeding the loneliness with tea and biscuits. And looking back it was easy to see over the years why I had slipped.

For me, the crunch came soon after. I was getting nearer to fifty and finding it hard to breathe deeply, almost all of the time. I was climbing over stiles whilst dog walking, or doing certain yoga positions, and finding I couldn't breathe in at all, whilst bending my knees up to my chest. Something was wrong inside my body and I didn't like it. Looking back now, I'm sure I had the start of a condition called Fatty Liver. Google it, it's not nice. I'd got into the habit over the years of relying too much on sugar in my coffee, and packets of biscuits whilst alone late at night after working all day at my job, especially during the mortgage/depression years. And I knew it was time to change. In myself I was feeling much better – back working with 'my kind of' people, I had a different manager, who was brilliant and understood and really helped me settle back in to what was expected of me and what wasn't, and things began to fall into place. Except this whole sugar thing.

The bitter truth about sugar

Needless to say, as this information is all over the place nowadays, sugar is 'the other white powder' but just as addictive. We know we shouldn't eat it – any of it really – but we still do! There's a strange mental faculty which takes over if you become addicted. If you haven't seen and 'digested' any of the anti-sugar programmes which have come to light amidst all the new science about how dodgy sugar is – in all its forms – please do. (See resources.)

I was surprised to learn – from YouTube no less – that even fruit juice could impact healthy bodies in a bad way.

I believe in this topic so much, I did a whole blog about it – go to www.debbieflint.com and look down the first page to click on 'Aids to Cutting Back on Sugar'.

There are a whole host of extras to help you understand. And in my revised version of *Till the Fat Lady Slims*, I've pinpointed as part of one of the key principles that it's vital to keep learning, to do research and to observe your body afterwards. I now know I can have an extra something sweet now and then – but I mustn't do it regularly. That's why I added the whole thing about getting off sugar addiction first.

Then and only then can you truly listen to your body's signals. Then and only then will your body be able to function correctly. And then and only then can you look forward to a much healthier life – some of my ladies have even avoided Type 2 diabetes by changing their diet and exercise regimes and turning over a new leaf breaking the habits of a lifetime around sugar consumption. And I don't mean just the loose type you add to tea. I'm talking about fructose in fruit, cereals, simple carbohydrates and so on – do carefully read through the section on sugar later and see how it plays a role in your own diet – especially if you 'can't lose weight' or have plateaued. It's your life in your hands.

16. Macrobiotics, the Microbiome and the Monkey

*A discovery which totally changed
my life and my own health.*

In the next few years, just like in the early 2000s, I began studying. I studied this new thing called gut bacteria that everyone was talking about as the new frontier in medicine. I discovered the Inner Chimp, thanks to a UK professor and his enlightening explanation about why on earth we do what we know we mustn't do! And I had another major Aha moment – somehow or other, I'd become intolerant of dairy. It was probably to do with the gut bacteria, or a lactose enzyme or something – I still don't know for sure. But I know things weren't right in my body and, determined not to be one of those fat and fifty-somethings, I embarked upon another major metamorphosis, starting with macrobiotics.

And I realised how differently certain personalities deal with the challenges of dieting as my foray into social media created an instant online support group – a supportive environment turning out lesson after lesson – and revealing to me something very interesting. I observed six main 'guises' of Freedom Eater (see later) all using different methods of incorporating the Freedom Eating principles into their lives. More than that, some of them exhibited a pattern of behaviour which I began to realise had affected me too.

The Wayside
I'd had certain periods of my life where I'd taken to Freedom Eating like a fat duck to Penta Water. And others where I'd been taken over by 'life', lost touch with my body and experienced what

we came to call 'The Wayside'. As in, 'We all visit the Wayside from time to time, just don't set up camp there.'

Listening to others, I found the length of time they each spent at the wayside varied, as did its subsequent impact on how guilty that person felt afterwards. This often included punishing themselves with self-sabotage habits. The six different types were even more distinct.

And something clicked.

I realised with pride that these ladies were all supporting each other to such an extent that the group took on its own volition and became a truly vital part of whether some of them succeeded in letting go of Food Prison sooner rather than later. A solid support system, it seems, was fundamental to long-term success.

But all this advice online, mainly on our Facebook group, and sister page, was being posted over and over again as new people joined. So by January 2016 I created the companion, book 3.0, with tips and tales to inspire, giving the profits to Medical Detection Dogs, one of the charities I support.

It all meant that Freedom Eating was entering a new phase, and it was based around having a deeper understanding of my body, of others' bodies and of how people are different.

Going back to my own tale, it was a massive 'Aha' that changed my diet more than any other as one of the Six Principles of Freedom Eating really came into its own. And it harkened back to that period when I was vegan more than a decade before.

Marlene Watson-Tara and Macrobiotic Miracles

A newspaper ad talked about a workshop in April 2012 in Scotland run by Marlene Watson-Tara (www.marlenewatsontara .com) where you learned how to cook yourself the best nutrition possible. So I went. And found a much healthier way of eating … of living … of being. After a couple of years spent expanding my knowledge about plant based, wholefood diets, macrobiotics and 'doctor nutrition', plus finding out about the foods my body didn't like, I finally accepted what deep down I'd always known – that my body truly prefers healthy food and hates others – in fact, one thing in particular, it really doesn't like. Dairy. I'd always been afflicted by a bit of asthma at certain times of my life but just thought I had a tendency to be asthmatic. Well, surprise, surprise, that thing I was so enamoured of, I had to give up as it was bloating my tum terribly and making me wheezy. Since then I've given up almost all dairy, most meat and much wheat, plus I've added essential elements from a macrobiotic influence. (See later – the 'Debbie-F (that's me) Plan'.) I was able to incorporate it all due to a laser sharp focus on Principle Six – 'listen to your body after you've eaten, don't beat yourself up, just learn and simply make better choices next time. Be an observer not a judge.' All in all, I turned a corner as far as being able to decline 'bad' foods.

I was also getting better at turning down 'bad' men.

I finished that awful relationship with the cheese-eating, cat allergy man, a whole 'nother source of despondency and baaaaaad sex! (He'd had a lot of women in his life – mostly one night stands though. In a little chat about 'technique' once, I questioned it and he said, 'No one else ever complained.' I said, 'No one else ever came back for seconds …')

So after that, I finally went back to full Freedom Eating, leaving the wayside behind. Only *this* time, armed with the extra information and resources I've talked about that helped me expand my understanding of the body and how it works, I was able to resume naturally interpreting my body's signals correctly and get Principle Six right. I reaped the rewards as my energy improved no end, just as it had all those years ago when I'd been vegan for three months. Plus I found my skin was glowing, I was no longer prone to feeling down and my taste buds got more and more sensitive, the cleaner I ate. Obviously all this healthy stuff meant my gut was very happy too.

Believe me, this gut thing is a revolution. I realised as I learned more and more, from people like Dr David Perlmutter ('Brainmaker') and Dr Giulia Enders ('Gut') and the YouTube video 'Gut Reaction parts 1 & 2' that there is a whole new world to be uncovered inside our bellies. And not just that, it also extends up into the brain via a connection called the vagus nerve, affecting emotions, depression and well-being.

Little did I realise, but by comfort eating rubbish and putting stress on my system, particularly as I got older, my body seemed unable to deal with it quite as well any more. The result was I was actually making myself depressed. Now you see how this fact might be stating the obvious? Only to some, as it happens.

Because others are still disconnected from the bloody obvious believe me, refusing to believe or see the results on their body and mind when they eat crap. Actually the ones who refuse most fervently fall into a category of Freedom Eater all of their own; I realised this type of person took longest to adjust to Freedom Eating, persistently overriding the normal signals from their bodies, insisting they could take or leave sugary foods whilst mentioning that they always have a couple of Magnums or eight pieces of fruit every day, for instance. It was an interesting time. I wondered what composition their gut bacteria took. Because every morsel of food affects the microbes in your tum, either beneficially or adversely.

Gut Bacteria and the Microbiome

So there is a whole new world in here! Inside our tums, there are trillions and trillions of organisms which affect everything our bodies do. But if you don't pay attention to your internal microscopic world, you might not have the health you would like. It amazed me to discover that some of the most misunderstood intestinal issues for certain sufferers being treated in specialist clinics could be solved with poo transplants – yes, really. And that my newly adopted beloved probiotics and prebiotics, fermented foods, miso soup and sauerkraut plus avoiding sugar or sweeteners, addressing the problems of antibiotic use, even incorporating new thinking on how a baby is born and breast-feeding, are all big topics of conversation in this new frontier in medicinal science and thinking.

See the further resources section later to be enlightened and please do read/listen/watch as much as you can if this type of thing fascinates you as much as it does me. It definitely helps you with Principle Six of observing and choosing more wisely next time, and of making those choices in the first place.

The biggest example I can give you is one about chocolate and sweet stuffs. I now know that if I have too much chocolate for too long, I feel down, and if I have a huge increase of it I feel depressed. Little wonder January was always a really hard time for me after a Christmas of elevated chocolate consumption – like most people, I'm sure. With a careful plan to wean myself off the nutritionally poor foods, along with a big increase in daily steps to help my gut, within two weeks I feel like a different person. Oily fish helps too, hence high dose omega 3 EPA being linked to lower incidence of mental problems. Do watch and read and listen to find out more, for example on www.fabresearch.org.

In a typical day I try always to add key extras, which help my internal community of good bugs to thrive – almost always miso soup at the very least, and a daily dose of probiotics – the more varied the better, apparently. Do your own research as to which are best for you. Again, if you can get them from food, great. But if you're on antibiotics, or if you have recurring problems with bloating or acid, google your condition along with the word 'probiotics' and 'microbiome' to see what comes up.

If you know someone with Alzheimers, IBS, or even autism, do read up on it all – for example the brilliant books by Dr David Perlmutter, such as *Brain Maker*.

And in relation to Freedom Eating, I realised that to give my body the best chance possible to emit those all-important signals, I had to get out of its way. As I discovered more and more about the crucial role gut bacteria play, I found myself voraciously devouring podcasts, audiobooks, YouTube videos and talks to help me really 'get it' and consequently to address it once and for all.

As a result of all this, and of my macrobiotic years, I realised how vital it was to add certain things into my diet that really make a difference. When I took them, I felt back to myself again. When I didn't take them and fell into bad patterns due to stress or 'life', I began to feel low again, lethargic and pessimistic.

So what's my ideal?

Probiotics, number one. Omega three, in the form of high dose EPA from fish oils. Other fermented foods including miso soup, sauerkraut, kombucha and apple-cider-vinegar diluted in water. Within about two weeks these have an amazing effect on me. The wayside comes along from time to time, but the beauty of Freedom Eating is that Principle Six clicks in if I allow myself to settle back into my body's preferred way of being. And if I needed reinforcement? Being an observer not a judge comes into its own. And the more I learned about gut bacteria, the more I realised this.

Something struck me. I looked back and noticed how quickly the demon sugar takes over again and that once it's got its claws in me, I find myself choosing less accurately at the next mealtime. And if it happens for long enough, I'll start feeling down. I know now that if I truly stop and listen, it's not body hunger that accompanies the cravings to eat crap. It might be an addiction, sugar being one offender, and fatty chips, crisps, pies, etc., being another.

So what is it that makes me do it in the first place, knowing I shouldn't? What is it that makes any of us do what we shouldn't?

Turns out The Chimp Paradox came along just at the right time ...

Making Peace with the Monkey

The ideal also means making peace with that Inner Chimp. And finding out about him was another revelation.

So there I was, thinking I'd got it all sussed, but from time to time slipping off and spending time at the wayside. Why? Turns out we need reinforcement. Reinforcement makes me determined and strong-willed. But being strong-willed sometimes backfires.

I'd always found the old adage applied to me over and over in my life – if someone says 'you can't do that,' I want to prove them wrong. If I try to diet, I know that as soon as the brakes come on, if I'm told I can't have it, I want it, even if I didn't want it before. To many people this will sound familiar, right?

Then there would be periods when I'd try to intellectualise my food choices – either to opt for healthy choices or even to try to do a diet, like a short-term juice diet which I agreed to trial – and found that I immediately wanted what I wasn't supposed to have. Even if I wasn't remotely bothered about eating it before.

Some other times, another type of behaviour kicked in, when I could easily act like a naturally slim person and I didn't want crap anyway, and making healthy choices came naturally.

I just thought that was me, that's how I was. And others definitely identified with that and told me they were the same. 'I know what to do but don't do what I know,' yet every rational cell in my head knows. So why do 'I' do the opposite? Why?

When I read all about The Chimp part of our brains, which kicks in when the 'human' part can't be in charge, it all suddenly made sense.

It's something I then wrote about in the companion book, *Till the Fat Lady Slims 3.0 – Tips and Tales to Inspire*, as it magically completed a part of the jigsaw that I'd always wondered about.

Turns out it's my Inner Chimp. There's a part of our ancient brains that was in charge when we were evolving – it faced life or death situations every day and its actions kept us alive. It's called the chimp, according to author Professor Steve Peters in *The Chimp Paradox*, and it makes us do things that seem irrational in this day and age.

When I read all about the chimp, I had another big Aha moment. I knew there was an element of my own behaviour I couldn't explain – most of us have it – and here's an example. My Inner Chimp inside my brain keeps biting off my gel manicure when the edge of the nail is snagged, like when I'm engrossed in watching a film at the cinema, nibbling and picking till it's all off, despite knowing that I shouldn't and it will damage my nail plate.

It is my Inner Chimp, which is also responsible for staying up till 4a.m. doing stupid needless things when really I should be in bed. It's the Inner Chimp's fault that I am often delayed and slightly late – consistently, efficiently, fifteen minutes late, to meet family, for instance. And it's the Inner Chimp that – very occasionally – forgets or overlooks or overrides the sensible part of my brain, which knows I don't eat dairy, and instead accepts a portion of cauliflower cheese or quiche, knowing that by tomorrow I will be coughing all morning and tonight my tum will look five months pregnant.

What does yours do?

One of my family's Inner Chimps does things like drink past the sensible limit. Then the chimp totally comes out of hiding, takes over with awful behaviour and nastiness when she's drunk, only to slink back into hiding and leave the rational 'human' part of her brain to deal with the consequences. And the next day can't believe she acted so badly. Well, it was the Inner Chimp.

It's a fascinating topic and accepting that 'it's just the chimp that did it' means being able to exercise the 'don't beat yourself up' part of Principle Six even more efficiently. And to allow myself NOT to keep on and on with that same behaviour, instead regaining control faster, and spending even less time at the wayside. RESULT!

So I've told the gang on our support group about it because it's a never-ending learning process, that's for sure. And every time I dip into the wayside, I know it won't be for long if I relax and accept that soon I'll be back out of it again. The Inner Chimp will be back in its box. Professor Steve gives various techniques for dealing with it and explains how it's helped all manner of sports professionals, and celebs and ordinary people. It's a fascinating topic and it kind of completes the jigsaw in my understanding of why Freedom Eating works so well for me.

Doing 'proper' or 'full' Freedom Eating is what my body responds to most of all, and using all these tools, learning along the way to remind myself about how and why it all works, plus picking up new life-changing information will lead to a long term escape plan from food prison.

But doing it alone isn't as successful as having a supportive environment, and our flourishing online support system keeps us all focused. Come join us.

17. 'NSVs', the 'When' Diet and the Six Guises of Freedom Eater

I'd love you to come and join ...

Over the course of the decade and a half I've been practising the Freedom Eating principles, I've set up a superb social media support system for anyone who wants to come and join. The 'stay in touch' section at the back of this book shows where to find it.

Lots of people regularly 'lurk' in the background and that's okay. Many regulars post the most wonderful updates and you'll find some superb examples of what keeps everyone coming back for more, and what aspects of the group has helped people get through some of the toughest times. Just to share in a private ('closed' is the term which Facebook uses) group, to offload thoughts or get help with problems or make suggestions or post links to programmes and books and blogs, means many people are succeeding with Freedom Eating where they never have before. So do come join us online via www.tillthefatladyslims.com.

Plus, considering how I recommend doing away with the need to have the scales govern your life, we often hear about 'NSVs ...'

NSVs – Non-Scales Victories

Non-Scales Victories are the best way to note your progress rather than being tied to weight loss. Our lovely members report things like inch loss, fitting into clothes they haven't worn for years, being able to put old rings back on as their fingers are smaller, fitting into an airplane seat easily, being able to do boots up, being able to reach their feet again, or see past their tum. Some have mentioned the comments people give them, especially people they haven't seen for a while. Or how they are able to report NOT repeating damaging behaviours – some even discussing how Freedom Eating has impacted other parts of their lives. It's a wonderful habit to get into, looking out for things to be grateful for in your everyday life, as you go through this Freedom Eating journey.

One of my own biggest NSVs was having someone call me 'little'. I was with a new man (I won't say which one) and he said to me, 'But you're so little.' It wasn't an adjective I'd have ever have thought would apply to me, especially considering my own self-image. I'd got out of the habit of saying all those self-deprecating phrases, sure, but something deep in my psyche still held those reservations about my shape. So this was a revelation to me, and I held on to that feeling for many months afterwards, I can tell you.

If you've begun this Freedom Eating journey and are gradually breaking out of food prison yourself, relegating the scales to once a week maximum, or never, do try using NSVs – it really makes you feel strong!

The Six Guises of Freedom Eater

As I mentioned, I have noticed over the course of a couple of years of dealing with different personalities on our online support system, that some of them deal with Freedom Eating very differently to others. The ones that seemed to have the same methods of adjusting, learning, reacting and bouncing back could be categorised into six distinct types.

For me, nothing has ever worked the way that Freedom Eating does – for all the reasons I stated about wanting to do what I'm told not to. I blame the Inner Chimp. BUT not everybody can take that plunge and let go straight away.

The 'When' Diet

As I've mentioned, after writing the original book, I met some people who were incorporating elements of Freedom Eating to adapt their habits more gradually. And I chatted to my sister, Linda – a former slimming club leader – and she helped me develop a part of the system that can be used alongside any traditional diet plan – ANY – called the 'When' Diet. It uses the absolute fundamentals of my Freedom Eating system. If you're like Linda and prefer to work to a structured programme, though, and you love the safety and discipline of being given a set of guidelines about what food to choose from – this is for you. Full Freedom Eating works for me, and for her when on holiday or during stressful times. But to lose weight she likes to diet.

When I started writing about Linda on my Facebook group, I had another key 'Aha' moment when reading people's responses. Not only was there an alternative to me, called Linda, there were also four other distinct guises or personality types that began to shine through. As I read the reactions to posts, and monitored people's habits, preferences, opinions and responses I created six specific names for six specific guises – and I list them further down – which one are you? There really is something for everyone with this system.

> ▶ *To help decide which of these most closely resembles you, do read the following. Mainly for newcomers, it's to prove you're not alone.*

1 – An Elaine.
2 – A Linda.
3 – A Sally.
4 – A Julie.
5 – A Kate.
6 – An Anita.
Appendix – A Della.

1 – An Elaine

Me! I cannot diet. Telling me I CAN choose absolutely anything means paradoxically that I don't want it – food loses its treasure factor. Research has a powerful influence on an Elaine's choices. Some Elaine's get it straight away and go on to become evangelistic about this amazing new way of being free around food. Some of the biggest success stories have come from the Elaines.

2 – A Linda

So my sis is the original Linda. A Linda is someone who prefers to diet as they feel secure in the discipline of counting and reassured by a framework that gives them the feeling they are getting it right. The biggest challenge for a Linda is to get past the tendency to override her body, relying on her brain to choose the foods, quantities, and timing. Instead, once she realises the difference it makes when she becomes in tune with her body's signals, it's a revelation. Also look out for the book *Woman Food and God* by Geneen Roth, a woman who is very definitely a Linda guise, as she reports loving the discipline of being on a diet yet still used to binge until she 'cracked it'. Some people start off as a Linda but ease into being an Elaine as they get in tune with their bodies.

3 – A Sally

A Sally is angry – she tries new diets or methods of losing weight compulsively, and it may work for a while, but then she falls off the wagon and becomes resentful, declaring that the world is against her and nothing works. And doesn't hold back, spouting long and often. Sally doesn't have a lot of self-confidence, and has spent her life feeling not good enough. She comfort eats to extreme and may stay in relationships or jobs that don't serve her. BUT a Sally WILL get it, eventually, once she accepts that the wayside is part of the journey, and when she does, she transforms into one of the other guises as she starts to see long-lasting success. But on the whole she is willing to give it a try.

4 – A Julie

A Julie is a mostly slim person but has a fat person's mentality. Julie also may rely on alcohol a lot (see Della below). She is also possibly under medication and experiences a really tough time realising how Freedom Eating can dovetail into her life. She does a good job of making it seem okay on the outside, but inside feels worthless and has been made to feel that way both during her upbringing and subsequently. She is like a very severe form of a Sally. Sally is too angry to be depressed. Julie doesn't have enough fight left in her to be angry, she is too far gone for that. Julie will work best with Freedom Eating if she manages to separate the rules surrounding her medication or self-loathing from the rules of Freedom Eating. She needs to work out a way of allowing herself to do both rather than to use it as an excuse as to why Freedom Eating doesn't apply to her. Further, she needs to separate her body's needs for food, and go back to basics. If possible, a Julie has to separate body-hunger from her mind's demands to self-medicate with food or medication or alcohol. She needs help to realise that she can indeed trust her body. She loses track frequently and gets very down. Some Julies may seem okay to family and friends and indeed present a decent front by seeming to eat healthily; but then they secretly go to the opposite extremes – some may self-punish by doing drastic fasting, or fad diets which cut out whole food groups. Her body doesn't know whether it's coming or going and can't settle or give her the correct signals as it is being disturbed all the time. Her microbiome is probably severely out of balance. She is out of touch with her body's signals and needs to examine carefully the way her body reacts to food by sticking attentively to the 'When' Diet. For instance, she may not feel hunger like she used to – it may now take on different forms other than hunger pangs, like feeling a bit light-headed or faint or irritable instead.

To begin with, Julie will benefit from a focus on cleaner eating, making sure she is not missing out on certain essential nutrients, get her gut bacteria right and allowing her body to reset.

5 – A Katie

Katie started out with a set of beliefs about what she could and couldn't eat based on a lifetime of being told different things around food. She is one of the last to change those habits. She has always been okay – could well have spent a lifetime as a slim person and only got fatter later on. She has always corrected everybody else's eating habits and choices and seems very assured about what is 'right and wrong' regarding food. However, she was probably very addicted to sugar. Initially, she was determined to keep declaring that she 'needed' to have 'treats' and that she could not and would not give them up. She insisted on finishing every meal with something sweet like a dessert. She kept her stash of 'treasure' hidden or closely guarded and everyone around her knew they faced death if they touched it. She had *very* compulsive behaviours around certain foods. She preferred weight loss systems which allowed these sugary 'treats', in fact if a slimming club sold them to her she would buy up tons of them so she never ran out, or sat finishing a pack of three tubes of sugar-free sweets before the class even began. The trouble is, she didn't feel satisfied with the one or two she was allowed under her daily rations, instead she regularly 'broke' the diet by eating too many, then telling herself that everything would be different tomorrow, so she'd just eat some more of these treats now to 'make it worth it'. In reality, her body is addicted to sugar, plain and simple, and she just needs to get off it in order for her body to successfully give out the right signals.

6 – An Anita

Anita has to exclude certain food groups – e.g. she has a tendency to be diabetic, for instance. She must count carbs, or count something, and has a list of what to avoid and therefore the 'Anita' guise covers all people who have to exclude certain food groups from their diet. One type of Anita has to watch her intake of sugars and is either diabetic or pre-diabetic. She's been told to count stuff, which she does semi-willingly and therefore adopts many of the Freedom Eating principles but does not go the whole hog, does not allow her body to choose with complete freedom, as her signals are jumbled due to her condition. (Many people think they are an Anita but actually they are not, they are just addicted to sugar – see the guise of 'a Kate' – and if they ditch the white poison then they move out of this category.) Some Anitas may be multiple things – e.g. diabetic plus allergic to yeast which is then exacerbated by anything sugary. So a double whammy. But when she tackles both, and crucially adds more exercise, it works and helps keeps her diabetes at bay. One Anita in our group has even reversed her diabetic condition with such management. They dip into the wayside more frequently.

Appendix – a Della – a word about alcohol

A Della is an Anita who needs to address the problem of alcohol first. Some women don't admit to themselves that they are drinking too often and too much and are relying on alcohol just the same way as others rely on food. Della needs to get this under control first in order to adopt Freedom Eating as her body cannot give her the right signals without doing so first. A mild Della may be not quite so affected by drink – or believes she is not addicted and that she can stop at any time and does not have a drink problem at all, 'only other people have that'. BUT if they 'need' to drink every day – really need it – or think they can do without but if they look back, they are actually drinking every night; or find that if they are on a diet then they get super-stressed if they can't add alcohol within their 'allowance,' then maybe the issue of alcohol needs separate attention first. Actually, it's in the same way that sugar addiction bars Freedom Eating from properly working based on your body's signals. A paradox I know, but that's what Freedom Eating is all about – your own freedoms, not a skewed version, based on addiction.

See the 'how to' later in the book for more about Linda and the lowdown to using Freedom Eating principles if you've always been a traditional dieter and just can't break free just yet.

18. What do I do, Debbie-F (that's me!) Plan

It may or may not work for you – you have to find out what's right for you – only you know ...

It's vital to emphasise that *your body* will tell you what you should be doing, you just have to listen. Your list will be different to mine, especially as no two people's microbiome is the same and no two Inner Chimps behave exactly the same way. In any case, I'm an Elaine, and you might not be, you might be one of the other five 'guises'. Whichever you are, I hope you manage to exercise too.

Since I wrote the original *Till the Fat Lady Slims*, I've incorporated some fabulous exercise into my life, including Bodyblade (google it, it's amazing) for toning up, and keeping healthy with the help of stretching, yoga and dog walks. Plus a pedometer or Fitbit has got me regularly doing nearly ten thousand steps a day and now that I've hit menopause, it's even more vital. In addition, freedom from Food Prison opens another door – to Freedom Living – see later.

The idea is you eventually find what works for you, so if you're able to promise yourself and me that this is only an initial guide, here's more of what I do.

1. My Daily Musts
- Tons of fresh veg, salad, a miso soup each day, a stir fry with greens most days, sweet vegetable tea (see marlenewatsontara .com for recipe) to help combat sugar cravings, seaweed strips for snacks (from Asian section in big supermarkets), some nuts each day but not too many (don't want to overdo it with the omega 6 as it reduces the good ratio of 6:3 in the

body – google it), lots of fresh water (not tap) and my choice of supplements.

- I avoid dairy, most meat and much wheat. I do eat fish and eggs.

- I take high dose EPA fish oils (1500mg a day of actual EPA) plus Vitamin C, CoQ10 and a good multivitamin. But also I've been impressed with Imedeen supplements – between January and April my skin density went from 47 to 53, a ten per cent improvement! Amongst others.

- If needed, a green superfood drink eg Barleans Greens – a powder you take in water. Contains roots and shoots and berries and leaves and grasses etc. Or similar – tons available online. Once a day or as often as needed – more if under the weather.

- I practise meditation, I walk my dogs daily, reaching nearly ten thousand steps most days; and every night before I go to bed I do a three minute yoga stretch – a version of sun salutations.

- Plus, when I can, a choice from the following: I have stepped up my Bodyblade use, doing, at minimum, the ex No. 6 hip and thigh for one full minute most days, giving the last 15 seconds all I can – that's what really works. (Search 'Bodyblade beach' on YouTube.) Plus one minute on leg master. I love the rebounders too; and if you can get one, the Pilates Reformer is top notch. But even if you just walk on the spot in your lounge, that's fine too. I clearly don't do all of these things all the time!

- I only have me to worry about most of the time, and my Labradors. I'm lucky, I know, but my hard work is done. But worth mentioning that I'm at a lucky stage in my life where I can do all this. But even when I still had the kids at home I was still doing most of this, the 'Debbie-F plan!'.

2. Suggested Induction – The 'When' Diet, Freedom Eating in stages

Week One
Introduce the 'When' Diet principles gradually.
- Begin by giving your food your full attention.
- Try stopping at satisfied not full, as often as you can.
- Definitely don't feel guilty if you have 'bad' foods – think, 'Does my body really want them?' If so, have them but stop at satisfied.

Week Two
- Pay attention to being properly hungry – only eat at six on hunger scale.
- Continue to stop at satisfied, and aim to get it right.
- Experiment with what effect different foods have on you.

Week Three
- Now focus on food choices. Hold out for the ones which really sing to you.
- Ensure you're waiting till six on hunger scale still before eating.
- Ensure you're stopping at satisfied – carry a container around with you to put leftovers in for later when hungry enough again.

Week Four
- Put it all into practice, every day, rigorously.
- Resist the influence of others, get used to the new habit of paying attention to your body's needs.
- If you're brave enough, stop weighing yourself.
- Join *Till the Fat Lady Slims* Facebook group and report your progress! Leave a review for book on Amazon or Goodreads – thank you!

19. Where I am Today

I truly am a new me.

I do try to contemplate the healthy option whenever I can, and to be honest, having complete freedom to choose any food means I regularly take the healthy option, naturally. Especially when there's no 'wayside' visit in action.

Full Freedom Eating advocates having anything you really want – no food is out of bounds. We all know that healthier is better. But if you can break free from food prison, guess what? Your body will know what to choose healthily anyway. This system should get you to the point of being able to desire the healthier options without needing to check in with your brain. It's just that if you're in a position of being screwed up as a result of so many years of deprivation and control, or if you beat yourself up regularly about making the wrong food choices, then you need to let go totally, and maybe even go through a brief 'eating crap' stage, before you can start truly meeting your body's needs to listening to it.

So don't think you can use this book as an excuse to eat only rubbish for ever more. If you do, you aren't doing Freedom Eating. Just keep the book and its contents for when you're totally ready for it. Plus if you get your gut bacteria right, and then explore the whole Inner Chimp topic, you may adjust sooner.

As your body adapts to its new found freedom, and you let go of the old restrictive behaviours, all kinds of weird things may happen, including initial up and down fluctuations in weight and strange reactions from friends and family. Just acknowledge, let go, learn and move on. If it feels good, then do it, do it right, and you will definitely start feeling good – better than you have done in years!

In which case, I'd love to hear about it! There are some stories on my website and, of course, on our online support group, from some lovely people who were kind enough to share their tales. Please see the details at the end of this book, on ways not only to contact me, but also to find out about other resources, and further reading mentioned in this book.

And for me the learning never stops, the Aha moments keep on coming and I discover something new about how to manage my Inner Chimp or deal with a problem differently, every time I come back out of the wayside.

One final story for you. Having had a major house move in the summer of 2015, I found I was very unhappy in early spring. I couldn't put my finger on it, but my stay in the wayside was worryingly long and insidious in a way it hadn't been for a very long time. It reminded me of when I was depressed, in fact. I knew all the things I should be doing but just couldn't get motivated to break out of a little post–Christmas down period.

Turned out my little cottage was getting me down.

I didn't realise how much it was affecting me but looking back now, it's easy to see. I was still single, my kids were happily living with partners, and work was going through a stressful time due to a fair amount of social media trolling of QVC presenters. But I wouldn't have said I was depressed, just not feeling particularly motivated. All the things I knew I should be getting on with felt like a bit of a struggle, to be honest. And when our never-ending wet winter finally ended with a holiday to Gozo to a yoga retreat, I felt like a whole new person.

Not only was I in desperate need of some sunshine, the retreat's menu and activities meant that my gut got sorted out once more. It's amazing to me how the wayside can come and go depending upon how resilient you feel. So I came back replete with vitamin D (I was probably a bit deficient at that stage) and plans to continue the healthy eating plan. But after a couple of months back at the house I ended up taking a trip to the wayside and not properly Freedom Eating during a writing holiday to a beautiful venue near Bordeaux called Chez Castillon, where the baguettes was heavenly and even the patisserie was calling my name – and that never happens.

So when I got back I took a serious look at what was going on. Work was good, tick. Social life good, tick. Charity work, definite tick, it was keeping me sane helping to raise funds and spread the word about the amazing Medical Detection Dogs, who asked me to be an ambassador. But when an opportunity came up to visit a guest house and writing retreat in Devon called Retreats For You that was for sale due to family circumstances, it was like a lock clicked into place and a door opened. Having decided I might go ahead and see if I could get involved with it and move down there, I realised it was my home which was making me fed up. It was tiny, which should have been okay as it's just me and the hounds, but it was in a little lane in a sleepy hollow between high trees and the sunshine was gone by early afternoon every day. Plus a sixty-mile an hour limit on the lane meant boy racers whizzed by and with no pavement, every day just walking the dogs meant taking my life – and theirs – into my hands. Finally the straw that broke the camel's back was really, really, really rubbish slow broadband – I work a lot online and even downloading a newspaper onto a tablet took eight attempts or not at all and enough was enough.

But you know the funny thing was that as soon as I knew I was not going to be staying there, once the house move became a reality, that feeling of hopelessness and frustration went away and it hit me like a sledgehammer just how much it had been affecting me.

The mirror told me so too. The wayside this time, post-menopause, meant a thickening waist, even though the rest of me wasn't too bad, and my compulsion to eat cake or crisps was being fed most of the time instead of occasionally. The wayside had a tent, and I'd moved in, without even realising it. SAD, it turned out – or seasonal affective disorder – had a lot to do with it, due to lack of sunshine – I blame my late shifts! But the new 'Devon project' perked me up, a return to feeling more like myself and to full Freedom Eating continued the remedy and I pulled back out of another crisis successfully. Freedom really doesn't just relate to the food. I'm planning to run Freedom Eating retreats in Sheepwash in Devon at 'Retreats for You' (.co.uk) at some stage each year too, come join me.

For now remember that if it feels good, it's probably doing you good, and every big change starts with the tiniest baby step, so make one today. Read this book, dip in and out or from start to finish, but just read it. Read it over and over again whenever you need a reboot. Join our groups online, visit my website and get cracking with the Freedom Eating, whichever 'guise' you are. Try making some adjustments so your microbiome is happy, and you will in turn be happier too in my opinion. Plus, research your Inner Chimp and learn how to manage him, for a whole new way of being. And most of all, remember the wayside is just a pit stop – if you don't set up camp there.

Good luck with breaking free from food prison forever.

Debbie x

Part Two

Further Resources

In this section you will discover the basic principles of Freedom Eating and

- The 'Super Six' principles – in bullet points.
- Freedom Eating – a workshop.
- Using Freedom Eating with a Traditional Diet Plan.
- The Six Guises of Freedom Eater – which are you?
- What if my body can't have certain foods?
- Tips on sticking with the programme.
- The Diet Rescue plan.
- Doctor's Orders – the 'When' Diet.
- What if my body isn't giving me signals?
- Why Sugar Prison is the worst kind of Food Prison and why your body needs to get off it so you can hear its signals clearly.
- A word about adding beneficial foods into your diet and the difference they can make including fat v sugar.
- What to do if you go by the wayside – as we all do!
- Binge Management – I haven't binged since 1999 but wait till you read this bit, owning up to what I used to do.
- How to keep in touch and how to get involved with our support system – it's there for you – do come join us.
- References, footnotes and further resources.
- Finally, you'll find links to my website, www.debbieflint.com and www.tillthefatladyslims.com where you'll see the latest inspirational before and after stories too, plus any press coverage.

The 'When' Diet

By popular demand, and just in case you've turned to this section first, I've now separated out the basic principles of Freedom Eating so it can be used alongside any traditional diet – any.

I've called it the 'When' Diet.

It's the foundation of Freedom Eating. If you are a beginner, this is where you start. It transforms your focus from just a list of 'can't haves' – of foods to avoid – to place the emphasis instead onto listening to your body. It's a kind of a game. A game you play with yourself. You can't lose, or fail, or be wrong. You can only learn.

This is where you accurately pick the right time to eat, when you can eat the correct match for what food your body truly requires in that moment, and then when you've eaten it you observe the effect that meal has on you – on your mood, your well-being, your happiness. It's all about 'when' rather than 'what'.

Remember – and this is alien to so many of us failed dieters – there's no 'wrong' – there's only learning, honing, and becoming more accurate *next time*. What's more, with this system, 'next time' is in just a few hours' time – at the very next meal, the very next time you're six on the hunger scale. Knowing the reset button is back to zero very soon is vital – it's not 'start again tomorrow', it's not 'start again on Monday'. It's straight away. It's taking back the keys to your own self-imposed prison – your food prison.

▶ *Because it's time to break free.*

I'm listing the basic principles of Freedom Eating here, in case you've skipped through to this section first. Read the 'What do I do, Debbie-F (that's me!) Plan' and 'Daily Musts' sections for the full in-depth explanation, along with what happened to me when I first discovered it all those years ago – it's all there in the previous sections of this book. But this is the nuts and bolts of what to do.

It's not magic, it's common sense – but for many of us, we stopped doing it a long time ago. The rest of this book will help you keep doing it, and that's the main difference between this and other systems.

Also please note the important sections about sugar addiction – and spend time doing further research – since you can't trust a body that's addicted, and do pay attention to the sections about new gut science and the Inner Chimp too.

The 'Super Six' – the Basics of Freedom Eating

The 'When' Diet is all of these, except if you need to follow a food plan, you choose the best match from what's allowed.

1. Don't eat until you're at 6 on the hunger scale, when the signals will be clearer to you about what your body genuinely wants to eat this mealtime. Think of it like the fuel light going on in your car. Only when you're sufficiently hungry will you make the right food choices. You're not saying 'I can't have that food' – you're saying the opposite – 'I can have that food – WHEN the time is right.'

TIP 1 – It's not a terrible thing to feel hunger – hunger is your body's friend – 'I never got hungry once' isn't a great thing to say about being on a diet. Don't be scared of hunger. But don't leave it too long.

TIP 2 – If you can't work out what 6 on the hunger scale means, imagine a scale of 1–10 where you are hungry enough but not starving, that's when to eat.

TIP 3 – 'I don't feel like it now' is a good response if someone's offering you a titbit you genuinely are not hungry for – you hear naturally slim people saying this all the time when they turn down food when they're not ready to eat or they're offered the wrong thing.

TIP 4 – New science on the vital job of gut bacteria is heralding in a new frontier in not only well-being and treatment of certain illnesses but also in understanding the body's needs for a break between meals. It allows your body to do a little spring clean. (See further reading for links.)

2. Be accurate in what you choose – *try to eat when you can have exactly what your body wants. Really listen to the signals your body is giving you as you consider each food choice. Ask yourself a series of questions if you're a beginner – do I want sweet or savoury, hot or cold, rich or bland, crunchy or creamy … etc. Then really imagine eating a food – the taste of it in your mouth – the sixth sense about how it will make you feel. Some people even smack their lips and close their eyes at this point. The food that 'shouts' the loudest to you is the right one in that moment.*

TIP 1 – If you can't tell what you need most, or *everything* is appealing, you're probably thirsty, so drink a big glass of water (the purer the better) and try again in 15 minutes.

TIP 2 – It's okay to delay eating until later WHEN you can make sure you have exactly the right food choices to hand. Some people are willing to delay eating a bit longer just to get the food choice spot-on, as the rewards are so great (see The Bliss Point game, in 7 below.) Meanwhile a little of something to fill the gap is okay, (see the section on 'pacing') just try to make it as accurate as you can for your body's needs at that time.

TIP 3 – If you're on a traditional 'diet plan' this is where the 'When' Diet clicks in – but you just make your choices from the list of foods on your plan. Simply be as accurate as you can even within the more confined range of foods on your plan.

3. Pay full attention to your food when you eat. *Don't eat until a time WHEN you totally focus on your food – do absolutely nothing else. If you're a newcomer, this means literally do NOTHING else – don't talk, watch TV, read, or drive and definitely don't pick up the next forkful ready to shove it in your mouth. Take your time – almost like doing a food meditation. Focus on the food and give it your full attention.*

TIP 1 – If you're going to pick from the fridge at least pull up a chair! Best of all, sit at a table to eat your meal. Beginners can even take themselves off somewhere suitable to sit down undisturbed to eat their food alone, so you can pick up on the subtle signals your body is going to give you about when to stop.

TIP 2 – Chew each mouthful for a long time, enjoy every morsel. Don't pick up the next forkful until you've swallowed, allowing you to focus on what's in your mouth.

TIP 3 – If you're properly hungry, and have chosen the exact match for your body's hunger, be prepared for the taste explosion! Some people utter ecstatic 'mmmm' noises so sometimes that's good to do in private! Hehe!

4 (THE MOST IMPORTANT POINT OF ALL) **Stop eating WHEN satisfied NOT when full.** *As I said the first time I came across this alien concept – 'What, you mean you don't keep eating till you can't breathe any more?!'*

This is probably the biggest change to your habits, and is absolutely VITAL. Once you do this, you can say you are Freedom Eating. No matter what you've been eating, even if it's what you would previously have called 'bad' food, this is the one non-negotiable principle.

TIP 1 – The deep breath. This crucial point of satisfaction is often indicated by your body taking a deep breath. It's a breath of relief. It's like your body is saying, 'Ahh, that's better, thank you, I'm done now.' But whilst hunger shouts, satisfaction WHISPERS – so it's vital to listen, observe, learn, and play the 'When' Diet game.

TIP 2 – After the deep breath, the taste explosion may abate, your food's flavour may seem to change and become less appealing.

TIP 3 – Your attention may also wander at this point – before it, you may be silent, just enjoying the luxury of eating the right food at the right moment. You may find you can now listen to other people as your attention is done with the food.

TIP 3 – A fistful of food. The satisfaction point is likely to come after about a fistful of food: your fist, not someone else's!

It's usually a SMALL plate full. Beginners – don't be surprised if it's half the amount you're used to.

TIP 4 – It's okay to leave the rest – it really is. And it's okay to SAVE IT TILL LATER – till WHEN you are hungry enough all over again and it will taste just as good. Doggy bags or To–Go bags or a little plastic container with an airtight lid are worth using. Or put the food in the fridge covered up ready for later.

TIP 5 – Beginners, be prepared for funny quips and comments from those around you, but don't try to argue or educate others – they may be food prisoners and haven't got the secret that you have. They are still conditioned but you are breaking free. Be prepared to do battle with others who think they should control how much you eat or whether you are allowed to save the rest for later.

TIP 6 – This is a magic one – Just say, 'I don't **feel** like it now but I'd love it later.' That usually works a treat. This is where social conditioning must be ignored and you can let go of the learned drive to finish your plate. No one will mind. You've had enough and can give yourself permission to stop now, in order to experience the next stage.

5.   Aim for the Bliss Point. THEN play the Bliss Point game: the rewards are boundless. Imagine you are a detective, observing your body like a private eye. Watch out for the moment your body rewards you for giving it exactly the right choice, quantity and timing. Your body will be filled with an overwhelming feeling of happiness and floaty satisfaction, and a quiet calm. Science is showing that hunger/satisfaction hormones halt or fire off at this point – they need time to filter through so be alert.

TIP 1 – This is a freedom, a feeling of control, and it makes you happy. The food is not in control of you any more, you are in control of the food. Achieving this bliss point sets you up ready to do the same again for future meals. Once you're used to it, nothing else will do.

TIP 2 – Foodies will adore Freedom Eating because you never eat unless it's WHEN the food tastes absolutely heavenly. Every. Single. Time. It's like some sort of pleasure ride. Stopping at the right time, having eaten at the right time, and only eating when you can consume the right foods, that's the 'When' Diet. And it feels exhilarating. You may even get a rush of joy, realising that this is how your whole life can be from now on. No more feeling guilty after a meal, or bad or sad.

TIP 3 – If your choice doesn't achieve this, and the food just tasted kind of 'okay' then you probably didn't get it right this time. BUT don't worry, let it go. DO NOT BEAT YOURSELF UP if you overshot and ate a little too much this time. Just wait till you're hungry again later and begin the game again. Think – when is it time to eat? When will I be able to eat exactly what my body wants, and when am I satisfied? It's all about observation, rather than deprivation.

TIP 4 – Also do not beat yourself up if you had something formerly 'bad' – eg, chocolate or some chips. Things that previously made you feel like you'd 'broken' your diet and made you feel a failure. With Freedom Eating there is no 'bad', there's only 'inaccurate'. This is a different game you're playing now and as long as you're honest, and only eat between being hungry and being satisfied, and genuinely choosing what your body (not your brain) wants, then you're playing the beginner's 'When' Diet game. You just have more to learn.

TIP 5 – No more 'treasure foods'. The more you do this, the tastier real food will be. You may notice how much less appealing all those 'naughty' foods are if you know they're not like treasure any more. You're a step nearer to getting it right more frequently and 'winning' the game. It's okay, for instance, if you eat what used to be 'treasure' foods – now you won't panic and eat everything left in the cupboards. Wait till the next mealtime and start the game all over again – if you've not gone past satisfied, it'll only be a few hours away. Most importantly do not beat yourself up, or think you've failed. And definitely don't punish yourself for 'breaking' your diet plan by eating ten times what your body actually wants. Those are old habits, and the 'When' Diet means you can't 'break' a diet, you're just playing a learning game. Learning to trust in your body again.

6. Examine the way your body feels afterwards and don't repeat the same choices next time if it made you feel bad. This is where you become your own science project. Even if you ended up deciding to consume cake or chips or crisps or whatever, it's important to do the 'When' Diet and crucially stop when satisfied. Then listen to your body some more – listen anew to the signals in your body.

It's a game, it's an experiment, and you are the scientist, conducting 'choice and timing experiments' on your own body in a way that will change your life forever. There is no failure at this game, there are only more-accurate and less-accurate timing and food choices.

As long as you eat within the above principles, you can combine *Freedom Eating (Stage One): The 'When' Diet*, with absolutely ANY diet plan out there. ANY.

If this is a revelation, as it all was to me in 1999, then read it several times. Many people don't 'get it' straight away – take baby steps, gradually adopting the principles above into your life. If you've been getting it wrong for a long, long time, it may feel alien but it will happen – trust your body, it's a wonderful thing.

Freedom Eating, a workshop

Here is how you can finally get out of food prison – if you want to do it my way. But just do it! Here's a basic step-by-step guide with some extras to help you 'get it.'

The first thing you have to do is to let go. Let go of all the rules you've ever learned surrounding food. You know the ones: I mustn't eat now, I must eat this before that, and not too much of that. I can fill up on vegetables, however tasteless and stress making they may be. I can't have 'bad' foods, or I'm being bad. I must be 'good' and comment on everyone else's eating habits too, to help me deal with my own inability to feed my body just what it needs, in the right quantity, at the right time.

The first thing I want you to do if you're looking upon this as a workshop, and you like to follow a plan, is sit and write a little list of what you would be like if you stopped being controlled by food, or overeating a little but too often. It's genie of the lamp time – three wishes can be yours – the body and life you desire. Right now. Let your imagination run riot. What would you look like? How would you feel? What would you wear? How would others react to you? In which situations? (Remember the future-you exercise earlier on?)

Writing all this down, and in fact, keeping a little bit of a journal about your transformation will really help you remember how far you've come. Pretty soon, it will become so natural for you to eat normally, you'll forget ever being any different. So do give yourself some 'me-time' and write. Keep it safe. You'll need it later.

Now get out those photos. The ones you hoped would never see the light of day. The ones where some horrid fatty has taken you over, and possessed your body. You were going along quite happily, doing the same thing for years and years, and then all of a sudden there in the mirror was this plump person, and you didn't like what you saw. You're not one of the tiny minority of perfectly happy fat people who don't mind being that size, and that's fine for them, but not for you. So get out those photos, and make a little album if you want. Or if it's all been too much for you in recent times, and you haven't even allowed any pics to be taken of you, get cracking straight away. Take some from the most unflattering angles, wearing the most unflattering clothes. Just imagine being able to take a photo of this fat person in the lens, and know that they are on their way out – their control over you and your appearance, and your inability to get into that little black number from a couple of Christmases ago, is all about to go for good. *It's about to end. Your journey is about to begin.*

Using it with a Traditional Diet Plan – Being a Linda

This section will possibly be relevant to the vast majority of readers who need to diet in order to lose weight. It continues the workshop.

The 'When' Diet principles, incorporating the 'Super Six' above, can be used alongside any calorie counting, points counting, fasting or food restricting diet plan. ANY. You'll just have a narrower list of foods to choose from.

So – when you get to Principle 2, just choose what you feel like most from the food choices on your diet plan. You can still choose what shouts loudest to your body – do it as best you can, where possible.

And if it's not possible as your plan is a defined list of meals you eat on specific days, and you can't vary it, you can still do the rest of the principles – as follows:

1 – Wait till you're 6 on the hunger scale.

2 – Be accurate in what you choose: what's the best fit, right now from the list you have to choose from?

3 – Pay full attention to your food, do nothing else whilst eating.

4 – Stop when you're satisfied. Listen to your body and stop WHEN it's time. If a diet instructs you to '*fill up* on fruits or vegetables', don't. No one should 'fill up' – everyone should stop when satisfied – otherwise you're eating more than your body needs and it will get stored instead of used up.

5 – Play the Bliss Game – assuming you have some degree of freedom. If not, just ensure you do Principles 1, 3, 4 and 6.

6 – This final principle is the most vital if you're on a diet that requires restriction, deprivation and control – do NOT beat yourself up if you come off it. Observe your body afterwards to help future choices.

Using the 'When' Diet part of the plan, anyone who prefers dieting will definitely be able to incorporate Freedom Eating into their lives – after all, it's a mindset. And it's thanks to my sister Linda that it came about in the first place …

Where did the 'When' Diet Come From?

My sister Linda was the instigator of a new idea I had in 2014. Because she loves to diet, she had a problem with the principle that nothing was banned. This is what she said:

> **27th July – sister Linda Bignell – ex slimming club leader:**
> *I'd seen Debbie lose weight and become totally different around food. She wasn't obsessive any more and seemed really relaxed around mealtimes. Even Bradley and Lauren seemed different. So when my sis gave me her book I read it and felt liberated! Always a member of Weight Watchers I would count and weigh and often override my body in judging the obvious! So although I still weigh once a week (just can't let go!). I now listen to myself more. What does my BODY want to eat? Stopping when I'm satisfied … Being more active … Smaller plates and portions…! I reached fifty knowing I'm not trapped in diet prison any more. I take the best of freedom eating skills and combine it with healthy choices.*

On combining Freedom Eating with Christmas and holidays:

> *For maintenance, it's amazing. The biggest thing that it did for me was that it changed what I did at Christmas and on holidays. Rather than abandoning a diet and acting like there's no tomorrow, thinking, 'It's Christmas I can overeat,' I was thinking, 'What do I*

*really want, and if I want it I can have it?' It made it
less like treasure. Having it when I wanted it meant it
was preventing me feeling deprived or overeating – it
was making me stop far, far earlier and I wasn't feeling
bad. The usual chocolates tasted waxy and weren't
hitting the spot. I remember the first Christmas I did it,
I didn't put on so much weight as usual.*

*I now do the same thing when I go on holiday –
there's nothing that's out of bounds. I'm not thinking,
'Oh God, I'm on holiday, it's all inclusive, I've got to
stuff my face!' I'm having what I feel like when I want it.
And not obsessing about it. I often want vegetables, even
at breakfast time, so the buffets were heaven and I came
back for the first time without having gained a pound.*

*Therefore it could be a big part of what people do
when they've lost the weight they want to lose. That's
me now. For me, it's now not a 'diet', I call it my plan.
When I ran slimming classes, nine times out of ten, the
very overweight people were eating to compensate for
something that was missing in their lives. For them,
learning the 'When' Diet will be a revelation. They should
also not be scared of hunger – it's part of normal life as
long as it's used in the right way. It's certainly changing
lives. And I am completely in agreement about the whole
Freedom Living concept too. And I love the Inner Chimp
idea. I call mine Tracey (my middle name) and it's Tracey
who is responsible for picking off my gel nails when it
knows it shouldn't! Debbie and I have a laugh about this,
it so rings true about why we sometimes do the things we
know we shouldn't, and it helps not to feel bad and beat
yourself up about it for days afterwards.*

*What's more, and what's really important, is that
having been an instructor for many years, I realised
that Freedom Eating had what was missing. Too many
diet plans say, 'Fill up on vegetables' – why? Why fill*

*up on anything? Eating until I am satisfied, not full
and not feeling duty-bound to always have weighed
portions of rice or pasta if I don't feel like it, is what's
working much better for me. I hate it when diets get
you to plan ahead too far – eg picking what you will
eat on Friday even though it's only Monday. My body
might not feel like that menu on Friday. Too many
slimming clubs talk about 'being bad', which makes a
lot of people not attend for fear of ridicule or guilt. Too
many people think diets work, because they can stick
to them for a short period of time but then they come
'off the diet', and go back to 'normal' which means
living in food prison till the next diet. Well, I now
know that a naturally slim person never eats that way
– they just listen to their body. Fortunately, some diet
plans and clubs are now starting to adopt these ideas,
but I remember Debbie talking about all this more
than a decade and a half ago. So I use Freedom Eating
alongside a traditional list of food choices and I call it
being on a diet, as that form of discipline usually means
healthy eating choices and my body feels good on them.
I like counting and it works to make me drop a few
pounds when I need to.*

*I'm proud that Debbie has called the Freedom Eater
who uses the 'When' Diet part of the system alongside
a traditional diet after me. I'm a Linda – the original
Linda – and I'm not alone!*

Email me info@debbieflint.com for information on how to get a
full podcast of the chat.

So the new guises were initiated and the list of six was born.
The main two are the Elaine, that's me, and the Linda, who uses
Freedom Eating principles alongside any traditional diet – any.
Read chapter seventeen to find out more about the rest and decide
which one, or ones, are most like you.

What if my body just can't have certain foods?

One important note; it concerns Principle 6. And here is where all the new information comes into operation. Information that wasn't around when I created the first *Till the Fat Lady Slims* in 2002. You see, whilst you're learning to recognise your body's subtle signals about how to eat like a slim person all over again, certain knowledge may help you on your way. And it all hinges on Principle 6 of the Super Six.

- Help with recognising addiction.
- Using research as an ally.
- Tips on sticking with the programme.
- Doctor's orders – using the 'When' Diet as a safety zone.

If you 'need' to avoid any particular food, the chances are that if you eat it, your body will feel bad in some way.

Assuming that's the case, you may be amongst the group of people who react favourably to news and information. It helps you interpret your body's signals more clearly to stay on track.

I made a major breakthrough with my own body's needs when I discovered via a week-long cookery workshop that my body doesn't like dairy. And sugar actually gives me hangover symptoms. And meat slows down my system. That's my situation, it may or may not be yours. You may have other specific dietary needs. So I choose more wisely now I know.

What is your situation?

Everyone's will be unique to them.

The whole point about the 'When' Diet is that you can follow what works for you – only you know, based on how your body reacts.

But you have to learn to trust your body once again.

Recognising Addiction

But what if you can't trust it yet? If you're finding it difficult to stop yourself eating rubbish, eg you keep 'wanting' chocolate, your body may be throwing you a curve ball. The 'When' Diet Principle 6, means observe your body afterwards – maybe you're addicted to sugar.

That's where the new information comes in. There's so much now readily available online, or from an expert, or in newspapers and magazines. Filling your head with the right information can affect how you interpret your body's signals and the subsequent choices you make. Just like finding out that some sausages may be made with pigs lips, tails or trotters means some people never feel like eating sausages again, certain information in our heads can affect our body's desires for some foods.

Sugar is a problem all on its own, however, as it's been called seven times more addictive than cocaine according to some studies (www.fabresearch.org).

Ordinary table sugar is made up of half glucose and half fructose, and it's fructose, from fruit sugars, which is the problem. This is all new information, and has changed how I view the body's signals, because a body addicted to sugar will just keep demanding more sugar and the whole Freedom Eating process is hampered.

I advise giving it up – becoming un-addicted – and then you can more accurately read what your body is saying. After all, logically, we all know that no one should consume jelly babies and ice cream, milk chocolate and cake at every meal. But a lady in a sweet shop tried to do Freedom Eating by continually selecting from the huge range of candies at her fingertips and then couldn't understand why it didn't seem to be working. Another lady declared she was doing Freedom Eating and described how she'd gone and bought what she really fancied from the supermarket – a whole stack of cakes and biscuits – and slowly devoured most of them in the course of a day.

That's not Freedom Eating at work, that's sugar addiction.

So I offer you here a bit of extra research to help you work your way more accurately through Principle 6 of the 'When' Diet.

Using Research as an Ally

For some, knowing more about the body makes a big difference. I changed my own interpretation of my body's signals when I found out what fructose does in the liver (from a university professor's YouTube video), and when I learned how a third of all the fructose calories we eat is automatically made back into fat –yes, really! No matter what exercise you do nor what deficit you have – all calories really aren't the same.

Plus it also taught me how fruit juice can be VERY fattening. I'd been drinking a famous brand 'with bits' every day, slowly putting on weight and unable to think why – thinking juice was good for me. How wrong THAT was! Also from 'food cure' expert Marlene Watson-Tara, I discovered how simple carbohydrates (including chips, crisps, etc.) also act like sugars and create insulin swings that actually prevent my body from releasing fat – whilst insulin is in your system it simply cannot get in the fat burning zone. In addition, new findings prove that the brain reacts to sugar the same way it reacts to cocaine or opiates: we really are addicted. It all makes me want to step in and refuse to let it control me.

Rather, I want to take back the power and be in control of me.

This kind of knowledge helps battle against addiction intellectually – and helps you understand better how to fight back against insidious, unnatural, man-made ingredients which will grab a hold of you before you know it. In my case, a little of what I fancy does NOT do me good. Particularly dairy.

I knew my body didn't like dairy – I used to bloat up something chronic and have asthma after I ate it. But via internet research, finding out that nearly two thirds of modern humans, globally, have lactose intolerance made me be able to say goodbye to it more easily. And I was someone who previously declared, 'No way ever would I want to give up cheese.' But feeling healthy is so, so much better than eating cheese. I also found out via Marlene Watson-Tara and her macrobiotic courses that a plant-based, wholefood diet is the best thing for modern humans to eat in order to shed chronic illness and recover naturally.

Marlene took her brother's prostate cancer measurement down to a fraction of what it was, following a purely vegan diet along with miso soups, seaweeds, home-remedies like ginger compresses etc. Food is a medicine, or food is a poison – and it pays to know which is which. There's a wealth of information out there, like never before. Watch the YouTube video 'Forks over Knives' for instance, and make your own mind up.

And it's not good enough any more to remain ignorant of the glaring information that's come to light over the last decade. I saw a food programme where the mother said something like, 'Who'd have ever thought that by stopping little Harry having fizzy drinks every lunchtime and no more burger and chips and sweets, that it would have improved his behaviour so much. I had no idea what he ate was so connected to how he acted.'

I'm not saying the same techniques work for everyone – everybody's got a different story. But if the basics of Freedom Eating: the 'When' Diet – are taking a while to kick in for you, that's when it's time to 'go google'. I'm urging you to go discover what your own story is.

Tips on Sticking with the Programme

*I know what to do, so how do I
continuously, 'Do What I Know?'*

Look, we're all human. Even with all our knowledge, we still sometimes do stuff that's not best for us, don't we? It's only this year when Freedom Eating became my priority again – my fallback, my rescue plan – that I've lost the weight easily. Really easily, actually. And I've packed the Inner Chimp away, more often than not. As I explained earlier I found out there was a root cause to my pit stop at the wayside, and once I'd fixed it, I was ready to get back in the saddle again. So first move is try to work out what the root cause is, obviously. But it goes deeper than that.

You see, doing all this research opened my eyes to 'food as medicine'. So when I got to Principle 6 of the Super Six, and really thought about the effect of certain foods on my health, I found that it was just easier not to put my body through it. So it became easier to choose more wisely. And address it head on, whatever 'it' is.

I know, by observing my body post-food, which foods I can have a bit of, and which I am just better off avoiding. Why give myself asthma by eating soft cheese, or custard or a latte with normal milk? For you, you may find once you're paying attention that you notice a certain brand of bread doesn't feel so good for you. Or eggs give you constipation. Or the kids play together much more calmly when they don't have certain ready meals, or half a can of soup containing four spoonfuls of sugar.

And through it all, you do it YOUR way ...

My own way is that I'm not telling myself 'I can't'. I'm saying, 'I can', which changes the psychology. It means a food is not forbidden treasure, which means I consider whether I really WANT to eat it. And once the Inner Chimp knows it can have it, it's not in famine mode, panicking and devouring the very thing it's been told it can't have, then the answer is usually no, I don't want it. And with all this new-found knowledge the learning process never stops.

▶ *So, so many things are possible.*

And if all this seems alien to you, open your mind and your heart – because maybe, just maybe, you '*don't KNOW*'. An ex once said to me annoyingly, 'You can't help being ill,' just because he'd never come across the information I kept trying to tell him. He promptly kept eating cheese on white bread with thick butter, milky lattes, and staying at his brother's to look after the cats, then coming down with asthma attacks. Turns out he can't eat dairy either and is allergic to cats. *No Sh*t Sherlock!* Just because you've never heard of it – yet – doesn't mean it's not true. That's the reply to use, for many so-called health 'experts' who just haven't kept abreast of new findings.

There's too much information out there nowadays to remain ignorant of it all. Especially if you want to seriously take charge of your life. That's what it's been about for me – getting healthy as I hit fifty and making sure my next decades are energetic and free from aches and ailments. If you don't make time to be healthy now, you'll have to take time to be ill later. And I'm damn sure I don't want to spend my later decades being ill. Be your own science project, and do your research thoroughly, in order to wise up to what your body REALLY wants and what you're best off eating. And whenever you're feeling stressed or under pressure, go back to the Freedom Eating basics, because the 'When' Diet principles can help you battle through the difficult first few weeks of any 'giving up' procedure too.

Diet–Rescue Plan

In fact, if you feel a binge coming on, check out 'binge management' later in this book.

And if you've 'broken' the diet, use Freedom Eating as a fallback:

- Don't panic, don't beat yourself up, don't 'start again tomorrow'. (Principle 6)
- Do nothing – it's okay to just wait till you're hungry again. (Principle 1)
- If it works for you, analyse what happened and why you 'broke' your diet – it's all part of the learning process. (Principle 6)
- Just aim to begin again at Principle 1 and wait till the moment arrives and your body's ready to eat again. It may be a longer time to wait if you overate last time.
- Choose what your body really wants – even if it's from a more restricted list of options. And if being forced to choose from a restricted list is your trigger to panic again, then just choose from a wider range of healthier foods, if you have them to hand. If you don't, go get them. Give your body every chance to achieve a bliss point by picking exactly the right food. (Principle 5)
- When you're a little more comfortable again, drink some water.
- Don't have a Last Supper, just do Principle 2 and pick more freely from all the foods available to you.
- Stop when satisfied. (Principle 4)
- Revert to the 'When' Diet and know that you now have full freedom to choose, as long as you stop when satisfied. That knowledge alone may take the edge off your panic and tendency to disobey your specialist's 'diet' plan.
- Do the Super Six and get back on track with your 'diet' once the crisis has passed.

Doctors' Orders – The 'When' Diet as a Safety Zone

If your diet means you HAVE to avoid certain foods, what do you do? My answer is that you do all you can to stick to the advice of your professional.

BUT IF YOU CAN'T, IF IT DRIVES YOU MAD AND YOU CAN'T STAND IT, AND IF YOU FREQUENTLY BREAK THAT DIET and you know you shouldn't, that's where Freedom Eating kicks in as a safety zone.

Use it as a fallback to help you make choices that will stop you going crazy. But do it **if – and only if –** it means you will avoid having a binge and feeling terrible, creating a vicious circle.

- Use it as a fallback if it helps to minimise the time spent 'off the wagon'.
- Use it as a fallback if the bliss point Freedom Eating gives you means you can avoid feeling bad about yourself.
- Use it if it means you can get back on the straight and narrow pretty quickly afterwards.

If you're like me, the mere knowledge that you CAN have something means it's robbed of its 'treasure status' and you don't eat it after all. Freedom Eating is a safety zone – helping you stick to your prescribed 'diet'. This is how those on restricted diets may find Freedom Eating useful. (See also 'binge management'.)

But what if my body isn't giving me the right signals?

You might find you are one of the many, many people who are addicted to sugar. If when you try to decide which food to choose each mealtime, you're always craving a bit of sugary food at the end, even if that includes simple carbs like crisps or chips, cereals or bars with a high sugar content, fruit juice or even tons of fruit, you might be sugar addicted. As I said earlier, discovering that first video about sugar, long before it became such a widespread issue, was amazing.

Plus if your gut bacteria are not happy, you won't find your body is functioning as it should. Check back on the section which discusses it all, in chapter sixteen earlier.

For now, here's the chief offender when it comes to your body not giving you the right signals … sugar.

Sugar Prison

My sister arrived at my house one day. Her son Ricky was training to be an osteopath and had told her about a video doing the rounds. So I reluctantly watched it. And it changed my life because by now, I'd become a lot stressed and a little addicted and didn't even know it.

Fructose – it's a chronic poison. Or so says a particularly adamant university professor in a ninety minute recording of a university lecture that became a 'sensation' from around 2004. I'd been back at QVC a year, and I watched 'Sugar the Bitter Truth' the YouTube video by Professor Robert Lustig in October 2010. After the fourth time, I kept getting my loved ones to watch it with me so I saw it over and over till it sank in, I gave up sugar completely. That Christmas, Andrew, a guest from Gatineau, the beauty brand, gave each QVC presenter five small Champagne Truffles in a pack. I'd had a particularly tough shift on a charity day and having been sugar-free for about a month I decided I'd 'trial' eating one. Then another. And another and another and another. That felt okay, I thought. For a short while. Then after a sugar high, I had the most horrendous crash and unbelievable sickness and headaches – a sugar hangover – for three days afterwards. Three days! I'm not kidding.

Everything started to fall into place and I realised what was going wrong. During the tail end of a relationship going bad, when sugar started to creep back in again to my diet, I found myself giving in to temptation and without realising it, it grasped me. I had a Christmas of being quite big – and quite ill. Lots of migraines and lots of not being able to breathe very well. I found that at work (on air at QVC) on a kitchen show if I ate lots of very sweet popcorn or one of our kitchen guest Simon Brown's bowls of upside down sponge puddings one day, that I swiftly got dragged back in like a quagmire the next. My body was being taken over like a demon, and once I had a little, I began desiring a lot more sugary stuff.

So I went on a healthy eating workshop in Scotland and the information I learned completely focussed me on how to more effectively do Principle 6 – be an observer not a judge – and pay attention to how food can both cause as well as cure illness.

I learned about how macrobiotic eating could solve so many issues. Within a week I was breathing more clearly having given up dairy and excess added sugar, meat and simple carbs. OMG did I feel healthy after! Within a month my skin began to glow, and after having had progressively fewer and farther apart periods (close your ears guys) I then had three periods exactly twenty-eight days apart. Unheard of for me, yet it was happening – something good was clearly going on in my body.

Talk about Doctor Nutrition! Or Food Medicine. Whatever it was, my hormones were balancing, my biome was regenerating and I had no more aching hands and joints in the morning.

It revolutionised my beliefs about what is possible in an ageing body. Any ageing body. We can all make the best of what we've got. Some things cannot be cured, but some things can – if you only know what to do. If you've ever found a product that changed your life, think about how you felt beforehand, when you didn't know about it. If someone had told you the change would happen would you have scoffed at them? But now you know better, right? Well, maybe, just maybe, there are some things that you're eating which are causing the issues you have. And maybe just maybe there are some things you could start eating which could help prevent the issues you have.

For me, now, I only get aching joints if I eat 'crap' food – swollen knuckles in the mornings – symptoms of arthritis? Well, Dad had it, God rest him, so no doubt I would have it too. That is if I didn't eat what I eat, and take what I take (high EPA) and avoid what I avoid. Talking of which – see below about the information regarding omega 3 fish oils and their many benefits to the body.

There are other videos to watch which will help you wise up about sugar on YouTube. Just search the words 'sugar' and 'toxic' and you should find videos like these:

- 'Toxic sugar.'
- 'Is sugar toxic, a sixty minutes report.'
- 'Sugar the bitter truth' with Professor Robert Lustig. The granddaddy of them all. If you're having real genuine problems banishing your sugar cravings – especially if you love finding out information – find out about addictive fructose and its effect on the body.
- And go to my website www.debbieflint.com to the home page where you will find the link to my blog with the latest updates – Aids to Cutting Back Sugar.

It's worth a try – search the titles and watch them several times.

After all, you can't say it doesn't work for you unless you give it a go, can you? And once your body is free of the sugar addiction, you'll find many of the principles of Freedom Eating so much easier to follow.

A Word about Fat v Sugar

Here is some other information about diet myths you may still believe to be true – new information has come out about low fat diets and it pays to be wise.

Professor Robert Lustig is the guru of fructose-avoidance theory and in his 2013 book, *Fat Chance: The Bitter Truth About Sugar*, and on his YouTube video already mentioned, he also explains in layman's terms how the health advisors in the USA got it tragically wrong in 1982 when the FDA began the 'low fat' campaign; it should have been 'low fat AND low sugar'.

Since then, the epidemic of metabolic syndrome has happened – showing this advice had the opposite effect of what the FDA intended. Why? Because manufacturers taking out the fat were replacing it with sugar. Just because it's lower fat, DOES NOT mean it's healthier. Check the labels. Anything over 5% sugar content should be severely restricted.

That's not to say 'never have it', IF saying that to yourself means you binge on it. See Principles 1–6 in the 'When' Diet! But if you're being sensible and using knowledge to benefit your quest for better health and a slimmer body, it's worth investigating this research. If you're like me, it helps me not WANT these high sugar foods. And a funny thing happens – when sugar is out of my system for a while, the higher sugar foods actually DON'T taste so good any more. My body doesn't want them – and neither does my brain. Especially since I found out how officialdom got it so wrong.

Google it. Everything that's happened since 1982 could have been totally avoided. It still can, if you get high fructose out of your diet. For instance, Professor Lustig says fruit juices are a no-no – eat the whole fruit, since the fibre it contains is also the antidote. And don't eat too much fruit in any case. Fruits with high sugar and low fibre are going to make you put on weight and any diet which says fruit is unlimited, but doesn't differentiate between different types, is out of date.

The only place fructose can be metabolised is in the liver. A third of all calories consumed from fructose are converted into fat. No matter what else you eat or what exercise you do, it'll happen. His 'Sugar the Bitter Truth' video shows exactly how, for the intelligent students amongst you (it's an hour and a half long and features much bio–chemistry). Or, just read his amazing book to see why it's so vital to make the changes to your diet now. If everyone did it, it would take society out of this destructive spiral of burgeoning health costs, he says. And any doctor who doesn't ask you about your nutrition when you go in for many common major illnesses, needs to also study Professor Lustig's work too. In fact, in summer 2014, it hit the news that key medical experts were calling for GPs to be more educated in nutrition. About time!

People like Professor Lustig and his peers are revolutionising public awareness about food and how it can harm, and how it can cure. The information is out there – go google, people!

Other nutritional extras – Omega 3 Fish Oils

Doctor Alexandra Richardson is another expert to listen to in order to help your choices be more educated, which will make Principle 6 easier. She's the Oxford professor who did those very first Durham school trials on omega 3, showing how children with certain attention issues can be helped with supplementation of extra EPA (an omega 3 from fish oil). This created the massive boom in omega 3 products.

Now I'm not going to say 'take loads of supplements, they're the best thing ever'. Ideally we'd all get everything we need from a balanced diet. BUT IF YOU DON'T, let me inform you about some of the information I've discovered. Much of which comes under the heading of 'Principle 6'.

Some of it changed my daughter's life as far as eczema was concerned. I'm not a doctor, and this is not doctor's advice, but as it's a semi-autobiographical weight loss book, I'm continuing with my own story and journey of discovery.

In the mid 2000s my small importing company had migrated into a promotions company helping health food industry firms create marketing materials. One contract was for a fish oils brand. In the process I became friends with Dr Alex Richardson. She told me, as only learned-scientists can, about the massive impact on the body of EPA (and to a lesser extent DHA), both a type of omega 3 from fish oils. Her current findings have since increased – now she gives talks about the research showing how omega 3 (EPA/DHA) can help hair, nails, skin, eyes, the brain, focus, concentration, sleep, depression, ADHD, the immune system, cholesterol, blood pressure, inflammation of all kinds, the heart, pregnant women (DHA), children under 5 (DHA) etc.

Erm, that's kind of … almost everything, right?

So – I could eat lots of oily fish from a non-pcb, non-dioxin, non-mercury source (hard but not impossible) or I could take high quality fish oils, which I now do. (Which ones? A pure one with as high EPA per capsule as possible – mine have 750mg EPA plus another 250mg DHA, but liquids can be high too and there are always special offers so shop around.)

More importantly, so does Lauren my daughter, who suffered from awful debilitating eczema during much of her childhood. She takes it in high doses, (2000mg) every day. This, along with avoiding SLS (sodium laureth or lauryl sulphates) in shower gels, helps her eczema stay under control, having tried EVERTHING in her youth to no avail. When she was about sixteen, suddenly we had the solution to her eternally scratchy, itchy, red, sore arms, legs, and bottom-cheeks, and a life of being covered with thick creams each night came to an end. She literally gained her confidence back and blossomed.

I tell you – if only I'd known all that when she was four! Then I began more than a decade of trying every known cream and tablet and Chinese herb under the sun. I'm okay with SLS but she's not. And when she avoids that, and takes her high EPA each day, she's mostly on the straight and narrow, on the whole. This is her experience, it won't be the same for everybody. Information can affect your choices. Just be wise.

Dr Alex Richardson talks about people who have brought down both their blood pressure and high cholesterol with enough EPA, and the studies Alex showed me examined depression victims and violent prisoners as well as disruptive school children, all of whom were massively affected by taking enough high dose EPA. Arthritis as well, can be hugely helped by it, she said.

So check with your expert but then go google. And if the expert says, 'I don't know of any proof' then they simply may not know of it. There are many not paying attention to nutrition news, and just handing out old advice – and tablets – willy-nilly for all sorts of issues. Marlene Watson-Tara has amazing blogs about diabetes and some very serious illnesses, and the effect of pure plant-based diets. Also, that according to the World Health Organisation, the vast majority of some of the world's top serious illnesses are nutrition based, or rather 'lack of nutrition' based.

It really is a whole new world out there.

Pointers for the Wayside

'The wayside is part of the journey,
just don't set up camp there.'

There are so many diets or systems out there which make you feel a failure if you don't stick to it the whole time. Even people who have a strict food list for health reasons sometimes still rebel, despite knowing it will make their body feel bad. In an ideal world, we would all do what we know the whole time, right? But we are human.

This may be the first weight loss system that acknowledges we often go by the wayside. What is more, Freedom Eating gives you a strategy for dealing with it.

First, here's a summary of the points I bear in mind when I hit the wayside, for whatever reason. Second, below you will find the last resort – if you're still in the early stages of Freedom Eating and have decided to have a binge, how to handle it. Personally, I haven't binged since 1999. This is a system for life. Re–read the book over and over when you need it, as we all do. We can watch our favourite films several times, can't we? Maybe months or years apart, and still enjoy them. Well, it may be because the human brain forgets. So along the way, if you're one of those Freedom Eaters who reverts to bad habits, or who spends too long at the wayside, then re-reading the books, using the companion book 3.0 and the online support system, Facebook page and my website will definitely help support this new way of being around food.

And if all else fails, read the section on Binge Management. We all know we shouldn't, but what happens if you still do …

So if you're stuck in the Wayside, remember:
- Only eat when you're physically hungry enough.
- Choose exactly what your body wants, not your mind.

- Only eat till you're satisfied, not till you're full.
- Give the food your full attention.
- Think about what your body really needs, not what your brain really wants and don't repeat old habits.
- You can do this even if you're on a diet.
- If you want something 'bad', go ahead and eat it. Or maybe if during one meal, you end up overeating slightly, just don't beat yourself up about it afterwards.
- Be an observer, not a judge.
- Don't set yourself up to fail by having too many rules. Forget every old rule surrounding food.
- Listen to how your body responds to the food in your stomach and learn how to make a good match. Learn to trust your body.
- Don't forget the water thing.
- Keep listening.
- Accept whatever shape and weight your body wants to be.
- Don't let others, or your own thoughts, get you down.
- Stand guard at the door of your mind.

Consider which Guise you are, join the Facebook and online support systems, and realise you are not alone. Read the resources and watch the videos, consider the Inner Chimp and your gut and go back to basics and the Super 6 Principles!

And never forget – the Wayside is part of the journey, just don't set up camp there!

Binge Management

Breakthrough time! The system that recognises that we're human – this is your emergency routine!

If this is the first section you turn to, then you may be still in diet mode, you still have the diet mentality. Great, read on. This will be good. The next diet will be 'the one', won't it? Stick to it like glue, will you? Lose all the weight? Keep it off permanently, right? Okay, fine. That's the place you're in right now and I know how it feels. I've been there too. Your next diet will work and you're not quite ready to let go of the habits of a lifetime and that's understandable. Whilst many can, some people can't. So, keep this book as a standby. It's the 'break glass in emergencies only' handbook, okay? Tell you what, keep it just so you never have to use it. Like the 'fat day' outfit you keep in the back of the wardrobe 'just in case'.

▶ *Just in case you need it, here's your Freedom Eating guide to binge management.*

Of course you're not going to break this next diet – the one in the latest book you just bought, with 'that latest celebrity before and after' – the one your best friend lost two stone using, and kept it off – so far. But *just in case*, this is your Elastoplast or Band Aid to help cope, to help stick to it.

How about a method of having that chocolate/doughnut/fish and chips/pastry *without* needing to beat yourself up about it afterwards? For those 'you know you shouldn't' moments, when all else (reserve, willpower, logic, fat photos, tears, anger, torment, throwing up, tablets, disapproval, tut-tutting partner or mother) fails, use these guidelines to make sure you minimise your time in the wayside – to limit your detour off the straight and narrow.

> ▶ *It is damage limitation and it works.*

It'll give you a sample of what Freedom Eating is all about. During a binge, you've thrown away the diet rules anyway, so forget the diet rules and try this method. After all, you may like it so much it becomes your new way of life instead of diet/binge/guilt/binge/diet – we know the routine. Read the whole book – if you want to – for amusement only, or, for curiosity value. Or dip into it in any order you choose. Do whatever works best for you. Then go back to the sections mentioned in the advice I'm about to give you – there's much more information throughout this book. However, for the serial browser – the one who has all the books under the sun and has 'done' each of them, but is still looking for the permanent solution, try this. And if you never need it, this book can be a great present for someone else who does.

Damage Limitation

The Rules are driving you round the bend. You're at breaking point. Or you're just too down or emotional to diet today. Or you broke the diet and now you want to keep breaking it and eat the entire larder then start again tomorrow. STOP! Forget the usual pattern just this once – and do this instead, and if it's your first time, then do *all of this* if you can. After that, just follow the main guidelines.

1. Take a breath and consider

Pre-binge, just give yourself a second or two to consider what you're about to do. And I don't mean the usual 'berate yourself whilst still consuming the daily calorie requirement of a Canadian lumberjack'. I mean think about this place you're in. Give yourself a bit of 'me time'. Jot down a few sentences about how you got here – write fast and furious – get it all out on paper, whatever 'it' is. Now take a breath. Literally – a deep breath. Several if possible. Stand up and stretch a bit – your neck, your back, your shoulders, more if possible. You're about to enjoy some wonderful flavours and the decision's been made – so calm down, you don't have to panic. But you might need to move a little – your body's signals may be just giving you the sign for, 'stretch me a bit please,' and you're missing it amidst the imminent binge frenzy. It's 'me time', and you deserve it, so stretch out.

2. Now drink some water
A big glassful if possible. If you're dehydrated you need it, if you're getting all anxious and hungry, chances are you may first and foremost be dehydrated. Dehydration is what commonly gives me '*I gotta eat, I gotta eat*' panic. But what it really means is, '*water, for goodness sake!*' You're going to eat something soon anyway, just give your body what it desperately needs first.

3. Now write down your binge list
Write down in order, the binge foods you'd normally go for. What would you have right now, usually, and what effect would they have on your body? Abbreviate if necessary, but just think yourself through it for a second. Forget the diet, forget about kidding yourself that you're about to stick to any semblance of what you *should* be doing, and go from your past record. List it from memory if you can. Perhaps the last binge was recent therefore easier to remember.

> ▶ *If you still feel the overpowering urge to dive headlong into a binge, you just can't wait, go ahead, but try this technique next time.*

One of my binges way back when might have looked something like the following:

• Vanilla slice – fresh (sheer luxury – starving – tastes like heaven).

- Caramac bar – (childhood comfort connections).
- Low-fat crisps – (something savoury – not too high fat).
- Ryvita and low-fat cheese and cucumber, apple – (an attempt to balance it out).
- Milky Bar, the chunky kind – (tasted nice at first, then got less flavoursome very quickly indeed).

My stomach is starting to complain, I can feel the food in my stomach. The tastiness levels decline and I'm feeling guilty but not enough to stop. I'm starting to get to the 'vengeance' stage – taking revenge on myself for being so bad. I know I should stop right now and it won't be too bad. But my usual pattern is to now continue, partly in order to wreak revenge on my body for giving in and being weak, and anyway, I want more chocolate in my mouth.

- Twix – my favourite, usually. Although now I can't experience a chocolate 'high' as the hunger is all used up.

Taste buds pick up 'it's chocolate,' rather than, 'oh my God this is wonderful, how could I possibly live without this amazing taste in my mouth. I'm so enjoying this I wish I lived in a sweetshop.' I know this, but habit and compulsion makes me continue.

Feeling fidgety. Still wanting to eat. Feeling appeased but not enough to stop. Torment; I know I should. But I don't want to. I've fed the feeling but it's still there. Maybe I should make it a big binge and go out and buy something else. Wait – haven't checked the freezer.

- Ice Cream Snickers and it's hard work eating this one and by the end, I feel a sickly sweet feeling filling up my gullet.

I'm on a chocolate high. I feel a bit spaced out. I still feel fidgety. I try to concentrate on doing something else.

I resume previous activity but it doesn't last long, I head towards the biscuit tin.

- Bourbon biscuit, and I don't like Bourbons but they're the only thing in there. I eat half of one anyway. And I remember why I don't like them. I might have had too much chocolate. I will try something else to see if that does it, something nourishing maybe. By now it's not about the need to eat, I've gone way past hunger. It's about habit, compulsion, self-punishment.
- Slimming chicken and rice meal for one. I hate to waste an expensive ready-made meal on a binge, but feel my body needs 'proper' food. Chicken, rice, and a few vegetables – there, I have had vegetables. I can be virtuous. Everything tastes like cardboard. I leave a little and put it in the bin. Hah! I can control self and leave some food in the manner of a slim person instead of compulsively finishing the whole meal every time.

Who am I kidding?

I think it's over. I go back to activity. I definitely can't concentrate now as my stomach is distinctly uncomfortable, and in non-diet state. I sit feeling more and more angry with myself. I must really diet tomorrow. I will eat half my normal diet allowance to make up for what I've just done today. I will be starving and the thought terrifies me, filled with dread at not getting food. Imminent famine and starvation and deprivation. PANIC!

- Other half of Bourbon.
- Other bit of slimming meal for one from the bin! Shit! I am now truly disgusting. I have descended to the pits of the earth, along with other terrible people from history.

I have returned to the dreaded Willpower-Free Zone – it knows me only too well. It knows my weaknesses. It sends demons into my head enticing me with thoughts of even more sweet or high-calorie 'bad' food. I try not to succumb. I try diversionary tactics, whilst beating myself up continuously. I check my weight, just in case, on the off chance my metabolism has sped up mysteriously and eaten up all of the calories I've just consumed. I get on the scales. Aaahh! I have gone back up to what I was two weeks ago at the start of my diet. I get off, check the zero calibration and twiddle the knob. I try again. Aaahh! It's gone up another two pounds. I try the knob a few more times. The only acceptable result is when the starting position is minus five pounds. It must be my clothes so I strip and weigh myself again. I'm still virtually the same weight, and then I catch sight of my fully naked body, stomach distended with an assortment of unnecessary binge food, my waist has disappeared and I swear I can see another layer of cellulite forming before my very eyes. That does it. I go and get on slob clothes and cancel going out. I decide to stay in and 'make a night of it', ready to start again tomorrow. Videos and sad music at the ready and over the course of the next few hours, I gradually complete the classic 'major' binge by forcing down the following:

- Three big glasses of Bailey's with ice.
- Entire contents of a 24hr mini-mart visit which I drove to in midst of frantic binge-mode, ate the lot including the following:
- Marshmallow biscuits – four and a half of a pack of six.
- Viennese whirls – another favourite – ate three of six – everyone more difficult to stomach than the last.
- Honey roast peanuts – the type I usually avoid because they're too high in calories.
- Smoked mackerel – I had to avoid this when I was on an old-fashioned low fat diet – decided to take advantage of the binge and have one.

Now I feel really sick.

- Crusty rolls and butter – hoping for sponge-like effect to soak up the fat.
- Two tomatoes and four slices of cucumber – a token gesture, which fails dismally to make me feel better.
- Still room for another Twix and three more Bounty bars.

Yes seriously, this really happened. In around 1999. And after learning Freedom Eating back then I haven't had a single binge since.

What Does Your Binge Look Like?

Have you got binge-paralysis now, just thinking about it? NO? It's okay, if instead you're thinking. 'That's what I do all the time,' just read this book and start being kind to yourself. It may be immediate, it may be a few months or it may be over a year, but if you allow yourself to start living and let go of food prison you will get there. Everyone's different.

So follow my method above, if you really, really have to have one final binge (after all, they are ALL 'one final binge' aren't they?)

Or maybe this time you could just eat all the food until you stop enjoying it, and at that point, play the game of 'I will have it later,' because you can, you know.

Think – how do you usually feel at the end of it? When is enough enough? When you go to sleep? How about choosing to be in control of NOT feeling that way this time? Especially if you wake up just to get a few more calories down you whilst it's still technically 'yesterday'.

With me, a binge used to be less a case of 'in for a penny, in for a pound', and more 'in for a penny, in for a limited edition, solid 24 carat gold sovereign, set with diamond inlay, signed certificate of authenticity and leather gift box'. Extreme to the max. Rarely done by halves, unless a miracle or distraction occurred. I always viewed my binge as if it would be positively the last time. In fact, this was obligatory in order to accept the binge would happen – it *had* to be the last time – ever. It always made me feel worthless, and confirmed my suspicions that my whole life would be permanently on hold until I could get this weight thing sorted out. And it was all my body's fault, and it just couldn't be trusted. But having read this book, you know that's not the case – in fact, the opposite is true. If you give your body the chance.

Record your feelings if you feel like it. This helps you to anchor this rotten feeling at the start of a binge instead of to the end. What's it going to feel like afterwards? How much will you hate yourself? What's going to be postponed yet again through having binged and therefore losing a day's dieting? I once sat with a friend called Marion who probably had bulimia, on the quiet, and we shared our innermost guilt about bingeing. I owned up that this was how I felt ...

Anatomy of a Binge

At the start of a binge, you get that sheer relief. When you get up to go to the kitchen knowing you're on your way to giving in and 'treating yourself'. You've accepted that the diet ends again now, and you just need that treat in your body. You can justify it somehow. Maybe it'll be just the one snack, though, this time.

Then again, maybe not. The first taste is sheer relief. It's heaven. *Welcome back old friend.* The chocolate you denied yourself is now rightfully yours once more. And the pleasure is extreme. Not only pleasure that you're eating the food, but pleasure that you're doing what you want instead of adhering to someone else's diet and rules. '*I'll show them.*' Maybe it doesn't start out to be a major binge, but the pattern is hard to break, and off you go again, into the dreaded ...

Binge Funnel

And when the Binge Funnel starts to suck you down, my God is it powerful, and you just have to go with it because it's a well-trodden pathway. You're on autopilot, your body and mind knows where to go, and you are helpless in its grasp. Whatever else you can't do in your life right now, you certainly know how to have a good binge. It's the certainty and significance of it all. You know where you are with a binge. You're in control whilst deliciously out of control. Deeper and deeper into the Binge Funnel till there's nothing but black and no turning back, no stopping, no passing go or collecting two hundred pounds worth of junk food from the 24 hour mini-mart.

Then it ceases to be about having food.

It's stopped being about the pleasure of eating. After a while, only the 'taste-on-the-tongue' pleasure, and the, 'saying yes, not no' pleasure remains.

After that it becomes about self-flagellation.

Beating yourself up and punishing yourself because you're such a bad person. You're repulsive, no wonder men don't want you and don't find you attractive. Or no wonder you don't get that job you want, that relationship with your kids, friends or whatever, ad infinitum. You deserve to feel like shit. So eat this, and this, and that. Take that, and that. Force it down. Make yourself feel sick, you deserve to. Maybe you'll get round to throwing it up afterwards. Maybe not. Sure as hell you'll be back on the diet/famine – an even stricter one than before – as soon as a new day breaks tomorrow.

It's All in the Brain

From then on it's all about a battle in your brain – if you can't control yourself enough not to eat what you should, you can sure as hell prove you're in control by eating what you shouldn't, big time, and then it becomes a matter of repeating old patterns, sticking with your identity. It's a well-trodden path, remember? And then punishing yourself for eating too much by … well, eating even more. Till you make yourself feel ill. Really, really ill. Isn't it amazing in this modern world when there's so much that's wrong out there already, and so much we're capable of, that so many perfectly-normal-in-most-other-ways adult females – and some males – can bring on this self-inflicted misery? Whether it's food or cigarettes, or drugs, or drink, or sheer depression, it's all a variation on a theme – events that we bring about through what goes on in our head.

> ▶ *So if we create it in our head, we have to end it in our head.*

Unless there's a physiological reason or deficiency in our bodies (see Julia Ross' book *The Diet Cure*, and your own doctor), then we are all capable of ending it, and just like the beginning, the end has to start in our heads.

> ▶ *And this book may be the very first step.*

It's not impossible to stop it. If you think it is impossible, and that you have to keep bingeing in exactly the same way, even if it's your own unique way, with your own conditions, then it's because *you choose not* to stop it. Maybe it fulfils some need in you like certainty, variety or perhaps, significance, i.e., it's the closest you might feel to love at the moment, *connection with yourself* and a type of behaviour you know very well. There may even be a little bit of growth, as you expand the amount you can consume at one sitting, and even some contribution, to your own conviction that you truly are a bad person incapable of reforming. Six human needs, according to Tony Robbins, remember?[19] And if the diet/binge situation suits you because having those needs fulfilled is more important than breaking free, then imprisoned you will stay. The only thing you can do if that's the case, is just stop complaining about it! Develop a new set of beliefs and tell yourself what you're doing, your regular bingeing and the rules you have about the way you do it, is okay, it's just part of you. But then so is being fat. And for many people being what you'd call 'fat' is actually okay, remember. So what's it to be – you decide. Just stop whingeing about it. You make the choices, you bear the consequences.

▶ *Time to change?*

Yes, we can opt to keep thinking the same thoughts the same way with the same outcome every single day of the year for the rest of our lives if we want. If you do, then that's your choice too, and it makes you no different from the countless other non-extraordinary people who can't break free from their rules either. It's up to you. It's all a matter of making choices. But I'm not talking about sheer willpower here. No one is more against the whole idea than me, of sheer willpower being the only thing you need. Willpower's fine, but it's not the be all and end all. It's not the whole story.

The same people who stick to diets compulsively their whole lives through are often the same sort of people who do everything in their lives in the same rigid, strict way. That's not most of us, it's not me and chances are it's not you – so don't be surprised when dieting doesn't work. What we need to do is be sensible – go back to basics, back to nature.

▶ *We need to listen to our bodies.*

Our bodies have an important role to play in the way we live our lives, and half the trouble we've got ourselves into is because we started overriding these important body signals in the first place. So I'm *not* saying overcome your urge to over-eat and binge by beating yourself up trying to fool yourself that it's all about self-control, and that you're weak if you don't manage to stick to a diet/famine regimentally. I'm saying *do it the natural way* – the way the body was intended to be – a two way street of communication. And this means, be kind to yourself. If you're forcing your body to overeat, especially to binge level, then you're just doing a variation of the macho willpower thing and overriding your body's important signals surrounding eating, instead of listening to the subtle nuances it gives out when it's time to stop, or time to sleep, or time to exercise, or rest and so on. We just need to re-learn the language. But step-by-step, with the natural approach.

So the next step now in Binge Management would be to think about some of these signals, listen, and communicate with your body. First and foremost, is it time to eat yet?

> ► *Preferably wait till you're really hungry.*

This goes without saying as a part of true Freedom Eating, and if you're just browsing through and this is the first bit of this book that you're reading, then do look up the relevant section about being truly body hungry before you decide when to eat. Then you can go to the next step of Binge Management, the question of what. Or rather what *not* to eat.

Step one – Solution – stay on the rim of the binge funnel

Instead of being sucked downwards in a never-ending spiral, what I'm hoping to help you with is to accept that you need to change your pattern at this crucial point, before it's too late and you're too far into the binge to be able to break free. It's freedom of a more advanced kind to be able to step out of the box and take yourself somewhere else when in a binge frame of mind. Believe me, the liberation you'll feel will be enormous, the sort of feeling you get when you step on the scales and find out you've lost a pound or two when you haven't really even been trying. A good feeling. Something new! Be adventurous at this point in your life – when all else has let you down – it's not your inability to stick at it that's made it fail for you, believe me. It's the diet's fault not yours. Everyone else is going to stay stuck in the binge funnel for the rest of their lives, but you can be the one that breaks free, okay? You've got the rest of your life to go back to the same behaviour, so for now, just give this a try. Let me be your success coach, and help you through this period in your life, but do it all in your own time, in a way that feels right, and works for you, or don't do it at all. Okay? And then in the future at some stage, you'll look back at the period you've just been going through – however long it is – and it'll be like some distant memory. So assuming you're up for it, you're going to step up and take your life to its next level, and with the initial help of binge management, get rid of this demon thing that keeps messing with your head and consequently with your body. So what's next? Well, if you're dieting, and you're still convinced that's the only way to lose weight, but the diet starts tomorrow, here's what to do about the choice of food to eat now.

▶ *Think about what you really feel like most.*

Of course, there's much more about these topics in the other parts of the book, and they're there for you when you're ready, but in a nutshell, for the desperate person on-the-verge-of-a-binge, here's what you do.

▶ *Become a food detective.*

Go and get all the foods in front of you. All the foods you'd normally force down you, in this binge you're about to have. I'm not saying you have to eat the lot, and I'm certainly not saying you can't. I'm not saying you have to now count what's in each of them and limit yourself, by calories or fat grams or carbs and so on, exercising yet more deprivation and control before changing your mind and eating the lot anyway. No, don't count anything, and if you find you still want the lot, you are being given full permission to eat every single last bit. As usual. But since you're off the diet anyway, use this occasion as an important experiment with Freedom Eating. I'll talk you through it. So off you go. Go and get all the binge foods. Don't underestimate it either. I want you to get every single type of food you'd normally eat. If they need preparation, just bring them as they are – still boxed if there's a picture on the box. That'll work almost as well. If it's just a pile of ingredients, it may not give you the right feedback, so do whatever you'd normally need to do with the food before you eat it. Unless you'd normally eat ingredients. In which case, bring them on! Now, with them all in front of you, I want you to look at each one, and work out which appeals to you most.

Step two – Virtual dining

▶ *This is one of the most important steps. Think about it. Feel it.*

If you want, do some Virtual Dining. To help you make your choices by imagining the flavour in your mouth, and what it feels like afterwards, thereby helping you to know which is the best one for you right now.

If you're truly body-hungry at this point, some things will probably shout out at you more than others. If you've decided to try it too early and you're not hungry enough, or maybe you've just had dinner, do it now anyway, and just pay more attention to the signals, then try to be hungry enough next time. Maybe tasting a little of each will help – the one your body needs most will taste the best. Some people will have laid out foods with a wide cross-section of flavours – savoury, salty, bitter, sweet and different textures – crispy, bland, crunchy, or chewy. Other people may just have a tray/table or floor full of variations on a theme, for example chocolate. If that's your decision this time, then fine. Another time see if you can bring in a bit more choice, as you'll notice the markedly different reactions your body has to the different types of food. Same thing if you're hungry – it'll make for better choices, and a better experiment.

▶ *Which shouts at you the most?*

That's the one to eat first. And the others in descending order of appeal. Forget balance. Forget previous patterns. For example, you always have the stir fry and vegetables first in an effort to fill yourself up so you're not hungry any more. Or you always have the steamed broccoli to feel like you're getting a balanced mixture and at least some goodness, or, you always binge on chocolate, so that's what you always have. Maybe chocolate isn't the thing that's jumping out at you this time. Perhaps it's the roast potato or the tuna soaked in olive oil.

> ▶ *Letting your body decide may be the turning point*
> *you've always longed for.*

Tell you why. When I first started doing Freedom Eating, one of the most amazing effects it had, pretty early on, was removing the 'secret treasure factor', from bad foods.

Step three – remove the secret treasure factor

You know what I mean? Every 'bad' food is like a precious booty you treat it like it's treasure, covet it, always want it even at inappropriate times, hoard it, hide it, want it in times of stress, use it as a comforter. Damn it, just owning it makes you feel better. You take it away on holiday with you or to an overnight stay just so you'll be prepared and just in case you feel you're going to need an emergency supply. But you often don't let anyone know about it. Because it's yours – your secret – your treasure.

So in a binge, you purely seek treasure, and load up on it, get as much as you can of it, in order to stock up and help battle the deprivation just around the corner.

> ▶ *But remove the treasure factor and those foods*
> *aren't quite so important in your life any more.*

And what happens when we can have something we want, without telling ourselves, 'no' any more? What happens when there's no restriction on something we've always deprived ourselves of? Well, you'll find out if you follow this process. But my reaction was, all of a sudden, 'Do I really want it then?' The answer came back more and more often, 'No.' or, crucially in a binge, not so much of it then. How many times have I started a little 'off the wagon' session, intending it to be just that, a little session, and ended up having yet another mega-binge, a Last Supper? You've done it too, huh? Well, if you can use the *TTFLS* principles instead to at least Freedom Eat your way through a binge, you never know, you may find you like the idea of freedom of choice so much that you want to carry on doing it this new way instead of ever going back to a deprivation diet again. If it doesn't work permanently then what's the point? If even a shred of you says, 'absolutely not,' then please do listen carefully to the next bit – this is where Freedom Eating gets really clever.

Step four – one of the Freedom Eating basics – do nothing else at all whilst eating the food. Give each mouthful your total attention.

End of story. No preparing the next bite. No reading the paper at the same time, just, take a bite, chew it, attend it, swallow it. You'll notice and remember every mouthful instead of suddenly finding all the sandwich has gone but you don't recall eating it, but no one else has done so, so it must be you. It's hard initially if you're conditioned to read/watch TV/drive/talk or cry at the same time. But it's only a learned behaviour. It really doesn't have to be part of your identity. Ever wanted to be someone else? Well, it starts right here. How can you get used to the idea of being this slimmer person if you can't even adapt a bit right now, especially when it means you can sit and really enjoy each bite of food? Believe me, try it a few times, and you'll enjoy it, get used to it before too long, and find it a comforting part of the whole eating process, and guess what? It's the way we were supposed to do it!

Step five – Listen for satisfied

Now comes the really clever bit in Binge Management. If you can stop the binge when your body has had enough food, sufficient food for the time being, even during a binge, look for the point when the taste changes and the flavour diminishes. If you can let yourself wait a bit before eating some more, and if you can try out the unusual notion that you don't have to make it into a Last Supper, then you'll be giving yourself a handful of true freedom. And that's not to be underestimated. Elsewhere in this book I explain more about how to tell if you're satisfied – an important distinction from 'full'. But basically, you should feel light and comfortable, energetic not lethargic, and you shouldn't be able to feel the food in your stomach, and you should have eaten maybe a portion of food no bigger roughly than a fist, and the 'drop dead gorgeous' taste will have dissipated. For me the biggest sign is that my body breathes a deep abdominal breath, as if to say, 'Haaahhh, that's better, thank you, I needed that, now I'm done.' I generally take a mouthful or two more, and that's it. *Please note I'm listing all this information here as a reminder, or for the benefit of those who have flicked straight to this section at the back – I know I would have. The full explanation is earlier in the book.*

Step six – it's all yours, you can save it and continue later

If you can't seem to stop at this point, keep telling yourself that all this food is yours, no one's saying you can't have it, just wait a little while till you're hungry again and you can have as much more of it as you want at that time too. Or something else that's not on the pile. Or forget the lot and go out for a salad. Or lose interest in it all because it's no longer out of bounds. Or find something more interesting to do instead, which may go some way to satisfying the real craving inside you. It's often not food we want, at times like this. It just feels like food-hunger, because we've always used food as the answer to every craving we've had all our lives. Or we've learned to later on. Habit again, see? But we don't have to be sheep and follow everyone else all the time. What about starting to discover what it is you really want right now. Is it hunger, really? If several mouthfuls of sweets didn't do it, and the same 'hunger' comes right back, then it's not hunger for food.

Fine if you decide to feed it with food anyway. You would have gone ahead and had a huge binge anyway, so it makes no odds if you do the same old thing again now. It's up to you. If you want to eat more right now, do it. But what if this can be the beginning of finding out what your body's really telling you? What if this can be the start of a beautiful friendship? A wonderful partnership? Rather than you hating it and not being able to trust it – or so you think.

Think about things from your body's point of view. What's it been feeling all this time? 'Silly brain – keeps overriding my signals. Told it time after time I don't want any more to eat right now. I didn't need those chips that time and I didn't need a potato right now – so I made it taste like cardboard. Why did my brain make me eat it when it didn't taste great, and the chicken, peas and gravy was what I really wanted, and some water. Still I'll be there for you, brain. When the rain starts to pour. I'll be here for you. Like I've been here before. I'll be here for you. If you'd only be there for me too …'

Step seven – go do what you're really hungry for

Or else, quit the binge – for a while at least – and go and find something that really fulfils your need. At one point just after I first started doing Freedom Eating I realised it was just a need in that moment back then to be held in my husband's arms. I loved being hugged. It fulfils some physiological need in me. I used to ache when I hadn't been hugged for a while. Sometimes I need a hug more than others. When I've gone without a man in my life and had that yearning, I fed the yearning with food for ten months solid. And ended up thirteen and a half stone. There aren't many times I've been that weight in my life and not been pregnant.

> ▶ *So thank God now for Freedom Eating. Because becoming body aware means I can recognise the signals that my body sends me and know that food,*

> *although a fleeting consolation, is not always the*
> *right answer.*

So go and find out what is, and go back and read the other sections of this book for more ideas.

Step eight – ongoing

Then become a food detective once more. You did it at the start to help decide what to eat, now do it after the food is bloating out your body to help make your choices, the right ones for you and your body, long term.

NB – this is vital. No one's saying that with Freedom Eating, you have an excuse for a perpetual binge. If you're not stopping at satisfied, and you're over-filling your 'gas tank', then the petrol is going to spill out of the fuel tank and into the storage area which are your hips and thighs and stomach and all the other places where your body stores its excess fat. And you cannot say you are Freedom Eating, 'cos Freedom Eating is stopping at satisfied. If you eat too much, you'll end up feeling lethargic afterwards. Your body is communicating with you, so listen, and more importantly, respond. If you can work out which part of the meal you just ate produced a reaction of wind, or a headache, or made you feel rather short of breath, or tired a few hours later, or whatever, then you are a food detective. Experiment. In true Sherlock Holmes fashion, work out how you can alter it next time. Have it with water, have the protein without the carb, have no mayonnaise, have brown instead of white bread, have more olive oil and start making it acceptable for your body.

> ▶ *If your body likes what you're giving it, it will let*
> *you know. If it doesn't, it will let you know.*

And if we can sort out the 'good for me' from the 'not so good for me' in that combination, it will save you masses of time in the future. Instead of trying all the different diet and eating plans under the sun, in the vain hope that a food plan designed for the masses can possibly meet all your personal requirements and also in the vain hope of finding one that may be custom-built just for your body. Instead, you can work out your own, by being your very own food detective. Then at least you'll be aware of the effect of your choices on your body, even if you don't particularly like the after-effects.

> ► *And so with a binge, try using Freedom Eating*
> *Binge Management to help cope the next time you*
> *feel a binge coming on.*

And one day, when you're through with diets, because you realise that they're only a self-imposed famine to which your body has to react to save itself from starving, by lowering your metabolism and thereby the amount of food you can consume without putting on weight, then you'll be ready to become a fully-fledged Freedom Eater and live your life with Freedom Eating, instead of in Food Prison.

> ► *And finally, binge–eaters ...*

So that's it in a nutshell then. Freedom Eating can help dieters through a binge as well as helping every other person to escape from their own particular food prison. The Freedom Eating girls are my saviours when it comes to 'falling off the path'. Don't think it's an overnight transformation – it's a 'getting to know yourself again' process, and that takes time. But it's bloody enjoyable. What? Yes, really! Imagine that every meal is a pleasure – a true pleasure not a forbidden one – because every morsel is eaten in a state when your body is ready for it, when you really are body hungry. It's given your total attention and enjoyed, as food should be. You stop when the flavour of the food diminishes because your body's had enough so it decreases the tumultuous enjoyment of each successive mouthful, and that tells you that you're satisfied.

Therefore you stop before you reach full up, overloaded, sick, heavy, lethargic, uncomfortable. For those reasons, every meal is total pleasure, never a chore or a punishment or something to be feared. Then you're following it up with an awareness process which helps you pick up yet more signals from your own physiology which helps you refine your choice-making next time round, helping you be a food detective and to communicate with your body in an ever-more sophisticated way. Eventually, you should be able to intuitively feel in advance what your body will feel like for every extra ounce of cereal you're about to pour into the bowl. You'll just know how much you need. And that means you'll always be one big happy bunny where food's concerned, rather than being a pain-in-the-neck, same-as-everyone-else, completely un-extraordinary, weak-and-feeble, no willpower, disgusting-useless-good-for-nothing (or substitute other alternatives you usually use about yourself on a regular basis), every time you break the latest diet/famine.

That's all it comes down to, you know. It's all just a matter of unlearning the rules that have brought us to where we are now on the food cycle. Go back to basics. Break out of prison. Food prison.

And the next time you feel like bingeing again, pick up this book once more, and try it over again. The more opportunities you give yourself to do it, the easier and more natural it will be. So don't worry that you 'can't trust yourself' to do Freedom Eating straight away. Just do whatever you feel you should be doing – whatever's right for you – alongside a traditional diet, whatever. And use this book like a faithful friend in times of trouble. The one who will hold your hand and say, 'It's okay,' even through the toughest food-crisis, because this method is all about the long-term, not the quick-fixes, or the rules and regulations. Read the bit about the wayside, and remember, the wayside is part of the Freedom Eating journey, just don't set up camp there. Then your stopovers in the wayside will become less and less frequent.

▶ *You've had enough control and deprivation in your life. Now try a little freedom.*

▶ *One final proviso especially for the binge eaters reading this bit first.*

When you first find out about a system like this, you may get all fired up and enthusiastic – and well you should be – it's a solid common sense system, with its basis firmly in nature. But I want to say a few things now, as food for thought.

▶ *It won't work if you don't do it.*

Someone once said to me, 'Freedom Eating stopped working for me.' Why? Because she stopped using it, and had gone back to dieting/failing/start again tomorrow. If that's your choice too, then fine. But re-read the book if you start to get lost along the way. They say we should do something at least twenty times, or for a good four weeks, before it becomes a habit, and feels 'normal'. The same is true of Freedom Eating. But once you do learn it, my God is it a turnaround in your life and if I can do it, *believe me* you can too.

Since changing my life with Freedom Eating in 1999, I haven't binged once. I've actually been mainly keeping myself out of food prison, even though the weight can go up and down, I just bring myself gently back to the basics, re-read the book, think about the principles and feel 'normal' once again. If you stick to Freedom Eating all the time, you'll keep the weight off so easily you'll think there's a catch. And if you knew what I've been through in the last three years, that's an amazing feat. And, yes, sure I've had little lapses into a little comfort eating, but they're little ones and they're soon rectified. In fact, what happened to me in one year alone (2001 – divorce, job and house changes, kids changing school etc) would have definitely made me comfort eat my way to at least an extra stone and a half, had I not had this system to rely on and get me back on the straight and narrow. Let alone what happened later! All related in this book if you're curious and not read previous chapters.

For now, you know enough to get you going on one of the most amazing life-changing systems I've ever known. And in all my years, I've seen a lot of systems!

You just have to learn to trust yourself. Trust your body's messages, maybe for the first time ever. If you don't try, you'll never know – and what have you got to lose? Will it be another ten binges before you decide to give it a go? Or are you going to take the plunge right now. Go on, go on, go on, go on. Need more insights? Let me help you, Mrs Binge Eater! Let me give you a picture of what it can be like for me nowadays, as a food prison escapee …

I went to a reunion of my Piccadilly Radio colleagues after fifteen years. Stressful? Absolutely. The old me would have binged all the way there in the car, then made sure I bagged myself a good plate full of the buffet, including dessert and coffee. Then having survived the evening, I'd have gone back to the hotel, armed with a bag of goodies for a solo binge, which I'd have made sure included half the mini bar snacks, and all the coffees, hot chocolate and biscuits on the tea tray in the room too. Then in the morning, I'd have made sure I got up and had the breakfast I'd paid for, even if it meant having a cooked breakfast I didn't really feel like, and balanced it out with some fruit and yoghurt just because it was there. Oh, and a token bit of jam on toast into the bargain. And taken what I could with me, including the mini marmalade, even though it was actually apricot jam and would sit in the cupboard at home for two years.

That was the old me. Know what the new Freedom Eating – liberated me did? Because I was actually ready to eat on the M6 when I stopped for petrol on the way up to Manchester, I got a chicken burger and onion rings – no fries, I didn't feel like them. But I did feel like a bit of Twix, and that's what I had – the rest of it I put in the glove box for another time, and when I got to the party, I still wasn't hungry, so I didn't have anything. I really, genuinely didn't want it. Nor the breakfast the next morning. Just an orange juice with my friend Diane who popped by for a coffee before I headed back south to the kids.

Another time, I would've been at Sainsbury's supermarket by teatime, but now, and because I eat late, I can have a coffee, with a big glass of water, and be quite happy just sitting there with the kids whilst they eat their dinner in a restaurant. Amazing. The old me would have instinctively chosen to eat a meal … well, just because.

And at Christmas, I can't tell you how great it is. Just after I learned Freedom Eating I had the first Christmas in my life where I hadn't put on weight. No putting on a few pounds as a result of succumbing to *scarcity fever* that I always used to believe was an intrinsic part of the festive season. It was finally working. And no more bingeing since then.

The Path to Freedom Living

This system has been helping a lot of people overcome their lifelong battle with weight gain and to start leading a normal life around food. I've heard from so many who tell me not only are they losing weight but are becoming happier within themselves. Partially this is because it's helping them use Freedom principles to let go of the need to control certain other parts of their lives. One lady, Eileen D., told me how it had made her realise she had to stop policing her daughter's behaviour regarding losing weight for her upcoming wedding, nit-picking at every single meal whilst they were out choosing the dress or making arrangements. Also to stop targeting her partner for his food choices. Even down to letting go of the need to walk the dogs in a certain way, arrange her wardrobe in a certain way, and live her everyday life according to a fixed set of self-imposed rules, or ones she inherited from her mother, or her mother's mother, or the people around her as she grew up.

As you've read, I learned the Freedom Eating system in 1999, when it helped me lose 35lb, quit binge eating, and mostly keep it off over the next decade and a half. In its entirety, you let go of deprivation and control and trust your body to choose the right thing in the right quantity at the right time. Everything changes when you let go of the reins. Nothing else has ever worked for me the way the complete Freedom system does.

Finally, as you'll have seen in this book, it's the most in-depth yet regarding my own battles. I've dug deep into my memories to share with you some of the most difficult times of my life and how I got through it, personally, finally embracing Freedom Eating again to return to my ideal weight.

Because there's actually a seventh principle – and that is to do in life what you feel your body – and you – really need. From meditation to walking to cutting loose from relationships that no longer serve you. If we listen to that tiny voice inside us giving us advice, often it's right. I do hope whichever element of this system you choose, it really helps you get 'Back to You' – the 'you' you were born to be, before society, a lifetime of dieting – and fructose – intervened.

This was specially written just for my new generation of Freedom Eaters who love a personal story – there is nothing like it for identifying that you're not alone. Commence your own journey, now or when you're ready. And don't forget to leave me that all-important review at the end or contact me via my 'keep in touch' section!

I truly believe this book can change lives. Why? Because I have seen it happen – a lot. Even amongst the doubters – eventually. It's very reassuring to see and hear testimonials from happy people who now have a completely natural relationship again with eating. Especially ones who initially didn't get it and were sceptical about it working for them. If it's not for you, please pass this book on to someone you think may need it and let them know about our online support group.

Whether I hear from you directly or via a review, I'm always interested in feedback. After all, the next book may be inspired by you!

References

1. Keys, A., Brozek, J., Henschel, A., Mickelsen, O., Taylor, H.L. (1950) *The Biology of Human Starvation*, Minneapolis: University of Minnesota Press.

2. Freedom Eating – Program One (1997), The Seven Secrets of Slim People, audio.

3. T. Robbins, *Personal Power 2* (1996), audio and CD sets and www.robbins.com Robbins Research International Inc.

4. Dr Wayne W. Dyer. *Your Erroneous Zones* (1988), Time Warner Paperbacks.

5. V. Hansen and S. Goodman, *The Seven Secrets of Slim People* (1997), Hay House Inc. USA

6. www.tillthefatladyslims.com

7. Pearson, L. and Pearson, L.R. (eds), *The Psychologist's Eat-Anything Diet* (1973), Peter H Wyden Publishers, p 250.

8. Freedom Eating – Program One (1997), The Seven Secrets of Slim People, audio.

9. T. Robbins, Unleash the Power Within Weekends, London Arena July 2001.

10. T. Robbins, Power to Influence Seminars, London, Nov 2001.

11. Sims, E.A., Goldman, R.F., Gluck, C.M., Horton, E.S., Kelleher, P.C., Rowe, D.W. (1968), *Experimental Obesity in Man*. Transcript of the Association of American Physicians, 81, 153.

12. Bennet, W. and Gurin, J. (1982), *The Dieter's Dilemma: Eating Less and Weighing More*, New York: Basic Books.

13. T. Robbins, Unleash the Power Within Weekends, London Arena July 2001.

14. Louise Hay and Bernie Siegel, *You Can Heal Your Life*, audio, (1996), Hay House Inc. London Hodder Headline Audio Books.

15. www.TonyRobbins.com

16. Dr W. Wayne Dyer, *Pulling your Own Strings* (1990), Arrow.

17. www.debbieflint.com

18. www.TonyRobbins.com

19. T. Robbins, Personal Power 2, (1996) audio cassette and CD set, Robbins Research International

Further reading

V. Hansen and S. Goodman, *The Seven Secrets of Slim People* (1997), Hay House Inc. USA

B. Schwarz, *Diets Don't Work* (1995), Breakthrough Publishing.

Julia Ross, *The Diet Cure* (2001), Penguin Press.

Deepak Chopra, *What are you Hungry For* @deepakchopra – fab exploration of the causes of emotional eating and *Magical Mind, Magical Body* including in audiobook.

Escape the Diet Trap – Dr John Briffa – @drbriffa – more of what I've touched upon here, but from a doctor's point of view, and full of fantastic links to studies, research and science. Can you tell I'm a science geek?

They are What You Feed Them – Dr Alexandra Richardson – also https://www.facebook.com/FABResearch If anyone knows what your kids should be eating, she does.

Macrobiotics for All Seasons – Marlene Watson-Tara – @marlenewt – macrobiotics queen explains why we need to eat like our ancestors. Her website, including a fabulous sweet vegetable tea to help combat sugar cravings, is www.marlenewatsontara.com

Fat Chance – the Bitter Truth About Sugar – Professor Robert Lustig – @robertlustigMD (It's all about the sugar, people!)

Brainmaker by Dr David Perlmutter

The Chimp Paradox by Prof Steve Peters

Gut by Giulia Enders

Till the Fat Lady Slims 3.0 – Tips and Tales to Inspire – the companion book to TTFLS 2.0 and to this new updated version.

So do your research – go google. Also go to my website www.debbieflint.com to the Back to You tab, where you'll see a regular well-being blog and an archive that's an armoury of information including so many helpful studies or the www.tillthefatladyslims.com resources page.

About the Author

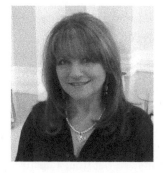

Debbie is a QVC Home Shopping Channel presenter. She started her career as the first girl in the hot seat on children's BBC TV, replacing Phillip Schofield in the Broom Cupboard. Then she shared a couch with Eamonn Holmes to help launch BBC Daytime TV. Years later, she hosted her own BBC1 game show (Meet the Challenge) and has co-presented and reported on numerous other live magazine and entertainment and news shows.

She is the author of short stories for children's TV (Buena Vista, 'Rise and Shine'), self-published fiction novels on Amazon and a contemporary fiction novel, *Take A Chance On Me*, published by multi-award-winning women's fiction publisher Choc Lit.

Debbie lives in Devon and has two grown up children and three feisty Labradors.

Follow Debbie on:
Twitter: https://twitter.com/debbieflint
Facebook: https://www.facebook.com/DebbieFlintauthorqvc
Blog: http://www.debbieflint.co.uk/

Links for this book:
Instagram – debbieflintauthorqvc

or Join the Facebook group 'Till the Fat Lady Slims'
https://www.facebook.com/groups/TTFLS/

and of course www.tillthefatladyslims.com

Testimonials

When I first started reading it, I was truly amazed – it was like reading my own story. Fast forward a couple of years and, to my surprise (conventional diets never worked for me!) I'm slowly and effortlessly approaching my goal of getting below the 11 stone mark – nearly 3 stone lighter. It's not hard either, now, as eating sensibly has become second nature! I love my new way of being around food and my new shape. But most of all, feeling normal around food.

Anne Keating

Being on crutches after always being a very active person all my life, was quite a shock. Weight had piled on. Then I read *Till The Fat Lady Slims*. It just clicked. No need to clear my plate, just stop when satisfied. Don't start until I am at number 6 on my hunger scale. I lost two stone last year even though I was fairly immobile. It's brilliant!

Sarah Hills

In 6 months I've gone from a size 18 to a 12! After lots of different diets (after being sick for 8 years and gaining weight) I finally found freedom eating. I read Debbie's book, then read it again and something clicked. I listened to my body, my body was not only letting me know when I was hungry (not thirsty) but also I learnt which foods suited me best, and about stopping when satisfied, NOT full. I didn't need 3 big meals a day, I didn't need a great big plate and I didn't eat just because everyone else did. The weight started to fall off me, even my rings are too big! The only things that fit me in my whole wardrobe now are my footwear, an expensive move haha, but wouldn't change it for the world. Thanks to Debbie Flint I now have freedom in so many ways.

Penni Rowe

I find freedom eating uplifting, and if you're a goody, you'll love it – every morsel at every meal feels like a treat. And getting out of the Food Prison trap of thinking 'I have to eat now', is truly liberating. Debbie's books have literally changed my life.

Hilary Ware

Have lost weight, gone down a dress size, look and feel better. Control my eating more thanks to the book. Have even taken it on my hols to read again. Best buy ever.

Christine Grochowina

Till The Fat Lady Slims changes lives it doesn't matter if you're able bodied or disabled, the principles apply. At the start it does take time and you do have to be brutally honest with yourself. I have been full freedom eating for 2 years. I might be a hare but it has become the norm for me now. Dress size when I first began was 20; am now 16 top, 14 bottom. Looking back at my old photos I look so bloated , my skin and hair is dull & lifeless. I feel so much healthier now.

Deb Sinclair-Bun

Till The Fat Lady Slims has changed my life so much, down from a size 30 at my biggest to a 12–14. Debbie's Freedom Eating system means I no longer have to panic-diet if I put a bit on, like when I disastrously went on hormones briefly. I just carry on with the basic principles from TTFLS & it slowly comes back off. The groundbreaking difference is that in the bad old days it would have ALL gone back on, as I beat myself up for being bad. This is such a life change for me, people who haven't seen me for a while don't recognise me, & I have to say I love it when that happens. Lol

Dawn Allen

I was a Yo Yo dieter for 50 years, going from 9½ stone to 18 stone and back, and have done every diet and slimming club on the planet. Then I read *Till The Fat Lady Slims* books I decided to take control, I sorted my sugar intake and committed to full freedom eating. I lost 12lbs easily, then averaged one to two pounds each week since, without feeling deprived. I am feeling so much better and loving being in control, it feels so liberating. I'm now around 3 stone lighter and delighted with Debbie and TTFLS.

Ann Swallow